I0425076

RACISM IN HEALTHCARE: ALIVE AND WELL

THE GREATEST BARRIER TO REFORM

MARIE EDWIGE SENEQUE, PhD, RN

IUNIVERSE, INC.
NEW YORK   BLOOMINGTON

Racism in Healthcare: Alive and Well
The Greatest Barrier to Reform

Copyright © 2010 by Marie Edwige Seneque, PhD, RN

All rights reserved. No part of this book may be used or reproduced by
any means, graphic, electronic, or mechanical, including photocopying,
recording, taping or by any information storage retrieval system
without the written permission of the publisher except in the case
of brief quotations embodied in critical articles and reviews.

The views expressed in this work are solely those of the author and do not
necessarily reflect the views of the publisher, and the publisher hereby disclaims
any responsibility for them.

iUniverse books may be ordered through booksellers or by contacting:

iUniverse
1663 Liberty Drive
Bloomington, IN 47403
www.iuniverse.com
1-800-Authors (1-800-288-4677)

Because of the dynamic nature of the Internet, any Web addresses or links
contained in this book may have changed since publication and may no longer be
valid.

ISBN: 978-1-4502-0800-0 (sc)
ISBN: 978-1-4502-0802-4 (dj)
ISBN: 978-1-4502-0801-7 (ebk)

Printed in the United States of America

iUniverse rev. date: 2/16/2010

To

Kate & Seamus

CONTENTS

PREFACE

Marie Edwige Seneque, the author of Racism in Health Care: Alive and well, has been a health care practitioner who has worked at various levels of the health care system for thirty years. She has worked as a registered nurse on three continents and among many cultures as a clinician, as a manager, and as an educator. She has a master's degree in Health care Administration and a doctorate in Adult Education Leadership. She was born on the island of Mauritius, educated and spent her formative years in England and currently resides in North Carolina. She currently is the President and CEO of a consulting firm providing education and management services to health care and non health care professionals and organizations. She is also an adjunct faculty member at the university of Carolina at Wilmington—School of nursing.

During a successful career as a registered nurse, Dr. Seneque started to reflect on her experiences and to analyze why researchers, health care professionals, and policy makers seem to understand so little about the power of culture and health and the disparity in access to health care access that exists among minorities.

Her diverse background prepared her to interact comfortably at multidisciplinary levels within large organizations, but she was always privately uneasy in her realization that many of her colleagues were culturally unaware.

During the four years of research for her dissertation she reviewed hundreds of articles and books on the profound issue of racial and ethnic disparities in health care. She concluded that racism was deeply engrained in the fabric of the health care system, thus denying minorities affordable quality health care they deserved. She decided that the truth needed to be unmasked for the sake of integrity and because the forty seven millions uninsured Americans needed an inside voice. She is not revealing anything new, merely compiling already existing data in a simplified, easy- to- read manuscript. This is Dr Seneque's first book.

The author hopes that the reader will find this book insightful and engaging and will obtain a basic overview of the health care status of disenfranchised Americans and how racism is a real barrier to health care reform.

The United States of America is a nation where people are not united because of those three glaring frailties: racism, injustices and inequities.

Yuri Kochiyama.

INTRODUCTION

In today's politically correct world, health care providers are debating and discussing inequity, inequality, and disparity but what they truly mean is racism in its many guises. Many health care professionals strongly believe that it is time to acknowledge and therefore eradicate racism in order to render the best possible care to those that need access to the health care system. The "R" word is avoided like the plague. Most Americans are very conscious of its connotations and the message it conveys. It is time to define the terms inequity, inequality and disparity so we can truly judge for ourselves whether health care professionals recognize them for the equivalent of racism. If they do not, it is because the huge amount of research published over the last fifteen years has focused mainly on disparity among our low socio-economic and minority populations rather than on racism.

In 1998, President Bill Clinton and Secretary of Health and Human Services, Donna Shalala, launched the Initiative to eliminate Ethnic and Racial Disparities in Health. This initiative, called Healthy people 2010, committed the nation to work toward reversing and eliminating the incidence, prevalence, and burden of diseases and adverse health outcomes encountered by minorities. Its very ambitious goal was to focus on and improve disparities in six main areas:

- infant mortality
- cancer screening and management
- cardiovascular Disease
- diabetes
- HIV infection/AIDS
- adult and child vaccinations

When this long overdue initiative was announced, there were kudos all around for work well done. It was a bipartisan initiative, which is a rare occurrence in Congress. In this book we will examine the extent to which progress has been made in meeting the goals of Healthy People 2010. A working group, on behalf of the National Institute of Health (NIH), was assigned the task of collecting data on African Americans, Asians, Pacific Islanders, Hispanics, Native Americans, and Pacific Islanders. Mary Lou Siantz, a former professor and associate dean at Georgetown University School of Nursing, has in various discussions mentioned that "NIH is trying hard to dispel these disparities, but it won't be easy".

Discussing the topic of racism in health care is similar to peeling an onion: there are many layers going deeper into its core. This book will try to dismantle and examine the many layers dealing with the very complex system that is healthcare. Physicians' attitude, nursing in the twenty- first century, lack of cultural competence, and the belief that the "R" word should remain unspoken must all be discussed as separate entities.

The overall purpose is not to rehash what is public knowledge about health disparities, but to look at each of these main layers of the healthcare system and expose how and why in racism is still alive and well in one of the United States largest and most costly industries in the United States. Although the United States is not the only country where minorities receive subpar health care, our focus in this discussion will remain in our own backyard. After all, health care spending per capita in the United States is much higher than in any other country, representing about 17 percent of the gross domestic product (GDP).

Experts agree that our health care system is riddled with inefficiencies, fraud, inflated prices, poor management, inappropriate care, and waste. A 2008 report by the Commonwealth Fund comparing the U.S health care system to nineteen developed countries found that the United. States ranked extremely low in the quality of care and had a higher infant mortality rate than the other developed countries. Money is not buying Americans the best care. Americans who receive the worst care usually belong to one of the minority categories, the elderly, women, and the poor. The causes are complex and rooted in contemporary and historical context.

Let me first define minorities. African Americans, Hispanics, American Indians, Asians, and Pacific Islanders are considered minorities in term of their race and ethnicities. Women, the elderly, and the poor are also minorities since they often do not have a voice in the health care decision making process and are stereotyped during the clinical encounters. This inequality of care has been well documented in various studies over the past decade and have been found in treatment of cardiovascular, renal, cancer, stroke, HIV/Aids, maternal and child health, and mental illness.

For a clearer picture, these will be detailed discussions although collectively the findings strongly support the hypothesis that race, ethnicity, and socioeconomic status are strong indicators of the quality of care that minority patients will receive. Rather than start with a picture of health care today, we will consider how and why biases, stereotypes, and even color blindness still prevails in the health care system.

We must remind ourselves that health care is not only one of the most expensive but also one of the most complex of systems. The current health care delivery system in the United States is undergoing revolutionary changes in response to society's demands for increasing access, increasing quality, and decreasing cost. Reform is necessary for the health care system to survive. There are certain sections of the American population that are fearmongers and will always find excuses not to reform a system that they know is crippling the economy and on the brink of collapse. In a political environment where key players very often answer to powerful special interest groups, discussions are anything but candid and the rhetoric is based on sound bites and seen through rose- colored lenses.

The Congressional Budget Office (CBO) has estimated that nationally as much as one third of health care spending is wasted and does not improve outcomes or render the best quality care. In 2007, one out of every three dollars that Americans spent on health care, or $730 billion, went to the insurance bureaucracies, drug companies, medical device manufacturers, and providers without improving a single person's health. Today, nearly forty seven million Americans under age sixty five lack health insurance and millions more with relatively good insurance lack prescription drug coverage or are but a pay check away from personal disaster. Young adults from nineteen to thirty four are the fastest growing group of uninsured, accounting for 40 percent of those without insurance. At the same time, prescription drug prices are skyrocketing, making it impossible for minorities, the elderly, and the poor to afford medications they so desperately need. It is often a choice between buying food or buying medications. As a result of this dilemma, patients who do not purchase their medications are labeled non compliant and not willing to manage their illness.

According to Shortell et al. (1992), health care delivery in the twenty first century will be characterized by transitioning from: (a) acute inpatient care to a continuum of care; (b) treating illness to maintaining wellness; (c) caring for an individual patient to accountability for the health status of defined populations. As mentioned by Peter Senge in his book The Fifth Discipline, "Systems thinking is a discipline for seeing wholes. It is a framework for seeing interrelationships rather than things, for seeing patterns of change rather than static 'snapshots' (Senge, 1990, p. 68). The organization's vision must not be solely that of the leader, but it must be created and shared with every member of the organization through open dialogue. "Team learning is vital because teams, not individuals, are [the] fundamental learning unit in modern organization" (Senge, 1990, p.10).

True participative and collaborative relationships in the health care system require a communicative, core-based ethic that understands self, valued personal experience, expressiveness, emotions, and empathy. Many health care organizations have realized that they need to include diversity training in their strategic plans due to the changing demographics and the importance of customer satisfaction. In almost all hospitals in the United States, workers and clients represent numerous racial and ethnic backgrounds. Diversity also includes socio-economic status, education, age, gender, disability, and sexual orientation. By clearly understanding our commonalities and differences, we can create a healthy and inclusive environment where people of different backgrounds can care and be cared for. But when we examine the bigger picture, racial and gender inequalities are endemic throughout our society. I mention gender because when researchers examined the inequalities in terms of gender, their findings were overwhelming: women of color fared much worse than their white counterparts in all fifty states.

In this book, the terms disparity, inequity, and inequality will be used interchangeably depending on whether our discussion focuses on access, quality of care or outcome. This should not distract from the core presentation of unequal treatment of minority patients within the health care system. "Racism is a hard word" says Antonia Villarruel, RN, PhD, FAAN and professor at the University of Michigan School of Nursing, "It means discrimination –the treating of people unfairly based on race or color that manifests itself in terms of attitudes". Racial disparities in health care and health outcomes are a disturbing feature of the American health care system and efforts to substantially reduce or eliminate them must be looked at truthfully by recognizing that such disparities are racially motivated.

Like most social problems, racism in America is institutionalized spilling over into a chronic and deep social problem. Although institutional racism may not necessarily be caused by intentional racism, it does however have very serious consequences. Jones (2003) is largely credited with explaining the concept of institutional racism accessible to the public health field. She very clearly sums up institutional racism as the result of the association of socio-economic status and race/ethnicity, via three main factors, mainly initial historical insult, contemporary structural factors, and acts of omission that occur when the structural factors are not addressed. these structural differences. Although individual attitudes may change, these acts of omission ensure that little else does, in part through denying an institutional role in determining personal health. We must first acknowledge that racism is indeed a problem.

Most white people are largely unaware of racism, especially their own (Trepagnier, 2001). One definition of institutional racism that embodies the health care system explains that "Institutional racism is that which, covertly or overtly, resides in the policies, procedures, operations and culture of public or private institutions - reinforcing individual prejudices and being reinforced by them in turn. Whereas individual racism is the expression of personal prejudice, institutional racism is the expression of a whole organization's racist practice and culture". Institutional racism is the major contributor to the disparities and inequities that prevail in the health care system today. Although less visible and more subtle than individual racism, it is nonetheless extremely detrimental to human dignity. Regardless of the fact that institutional racism is not caused intentionally, it carries disastrous consequences for persons of color in terms of health outcomes. We must therefore be informed by understanding the factors that underlie and contribute to the policies, guidelines, and practices that enable institutional racism.

Previous presidents, Republican and Democrat, from Roosevelt to Clinton have proposed ways in which to reform the American health care system. Along the way there have been small significant changes. But there has always been a huge roadblock mounted by those who benefit the most from a chaotic system: the powerful insurance and pharmaceutical companies. No administration has succeeded in bringing substantial changes that would benefit those in need of affordable and quality care. We should not focus solely on affordable health care, but quality of care as well. Inclusive health care is what is really needed in a just society. With the current spotlight on reform, now is the time not only to change a system that is on the verge of collapse and benefitting only the privileged class.

Do we once again spend billions of dollars to revamp parts of a system that is on the brink of collapse? If a house was on the verge of sinking because of the huge cracks in its foundation, it would be insane to hire an interior decorator to revamp the décor. The health care system has on numerous occasions received minor remodeling while inspection still reveals that impending collapse is looming large due to a crumbling foundation. What will our current president do? Will there be more Band-Aid approaches?

African Americans, Hispanics, Asians, Pacific Islanders, and Native Americans suffer disproportionate burdens of morbidity and mortality in the United States today. Yet most of us do not question why such disparity continues unabated. The time to provide all Americans with a health care system they deserve as citizens of the richest country in the world is now or never. With the anticipated health care reform, it is the hope of many that those lofty words from the Declaration of independence will at last ring true: "We hold these truths to be self-evident, that all men are created equal." However, a fundamental shift in awareness, values, and attitudes is necessary. The institutional structures that sustain policies and practices of ingrained patterns of inequality and exclusion must be dismantled.

To achieve health care reform that will benefit all Americans regardless of race and socioeconomic status, those who truly believe in social justice will need to build a broad based movement that cut across party lines. Americans of good faith, those without an agenda will need to tighten ranks so that the voices of the underinsured, as well as those of the uninsured and the poor can be heard loud and clear on Capitol Hill. Quality health care is a human right

Some may dismiss this as another book on race, or it may enrage many who would rather keep the closet securely locked. I hope this book will generate excitement and controversy and engage many in candid conversations about ingrained institutional racism and the existing racial inequalities in twenty first century health care .

Each of us shines in a different way, but this doesn't make our light less bright. Peace cannot be kept by force; it can only be achieved by understanding.

Albert Einstein

CHAPTER 1
RACE AND HEALTH

Thomas Jefferson was the first person to write about "race" when introducing the idea of an inferior people. In a country founded both on the principle that "all men are created equal," and on the economic base of slavery, the idea of "race" helped explain why some people could be denied the rights and freedoms that others took as a given. In the first census of 1790, racial categories were specifically spelled out as not being equal: blacks were only considered only three-fifths of a person in comparison to whites. The Thirteenth Amendment finally ended the three-fifths rule, and over time new racial categories were added to the census to keep track of new immigrants. Racial categorization is rooted in racism and our racial groupings capture important differences in power, status, and resources. Throughout U.S. history, racial classification has ranked the various racial groups implicitly or explicitly with whites on the top, blacks on the bottom, and other groups in between.

Racism involves more than just race and should be viewed as a system of oppressive ethnic and race relations. In this relationship, there is always a dominant group that reaps huge benefits by dominating another who is identified as inferior. Race is a social construct rather than a biological concept. Ideologically, racism is deeply entrenched in the socioeconomic and political realities of American society. Today, race continues to be one of the determinants of health allocations. Lack of education, lack of job opportunities, low socioeconomic status, and residential segregation are all strong social indicators that allow racism to still exist within institutional structures.

In 1800, seventy three blacks living in Philadelphia signed a petition that was sent to Congress. They asked that Congress debate for the extension of America's "promises" of freedom and justice to persons of color. They also wanted protection from the abominable practice of kidnapping free blacks and delivering them into slavery. Congress rejected the petition. The days of slavery and the treatment of slaves have been extensively documented and will not be rehashed here, but it is important to remember that in the early eighteenth and nineteenth centuries slaves were the property of their masters and as such had little say about their state of health and wellness.

The slave owners rationalized their domination in terms of blacks as being inferior and requiring close supervision for their own good. Slaves were therefore dependent on their masters for their health care. Despite the availability of care and the self interest of the owners to keep their slaves healthy, the quality of care for the person of color was below standard. Reporting illness often meant a reprimand for being lazy or at worst physical punishment. Fearing such attention many slaves treated themselves with herbs and folklore remedies. Self treatment and mistrust of available health care started during this period in our history and surely increased after the revelation of the Tuskegee incident. Then and now, self care often turns an acute ailment into a chronic debilitating one.

It is only fair that a brief overview of the Tuskegee incident is given as this was decidedly the start of the mistrust that still manifest itself today between the black community and the health care system.

The owners and overseers perceived the slaves as subhuman, inferior biologically and intellectually, and incapable of looking after themselves and their children. This conclusion was based on the construct of racial determinant rather than on the slaves' social dilemma. Slaves encountered confined living quarters, unsanitary waste practices, contaminated drinking water, poor nutrition, stress, and the spread of infection through bacteria and parasites. Blacks were also less tolerant of the harsh medical treatments of the time. The poor health of the slaves was therefore not due to their biological inferiority but rather their substandard environmental. In 1855, the Richmond medical journal declared that "the African constitution sinks before the heavy blows of the medical treatments that advocated large doses of medicines and treatments such as bleeding, purgatives, and emetics that depleted the body". We can understand more clearly how major racially structured institutions such as slavery, internment camps, and Indian reservations have produced their share of atrocities and unequal treatments.

Throughout the history of the United States, race and class combined with other factors have established a "slave health deficit". The worst atrocities and the very reason for continued mistrust can be attributed to the period of research when non consensual medical experiments were performed. Thomas Jefferson inoculated hundreds of his slaves with the smallpox virus to determine the viability of an experimental vaccine. Medical schools relied on the bodies of African Americans for cadaver research. Medical institutions hired grave robbers to steal newly buried bodies of blacks to maintain a supply of cadavers for their experiments. The most famous of all nonconsensual experiments happened during the Jim Crow era. The Tuskegee syphilis experiment began in 1932. Forty years after this experiment the surviving subjects were informed that they had been part of the longest non-consensual experiment and that penicillin, the known effective treatment, was withheld. As many history books and studies report, overt segregation in health care access remained intact until around 1964 when Congress passed the Civil Rights Act.

Although founded in 1847, the American Medical Association (AMA) did not welcome people of color doctor until the late 1960s. Despite minority candidates' pursuit of training in health professions, the American health care system excluded people of color as doctors, dentists, and nurses well into the second half of the twentieth century. In the early years of the twentieth century, racism was spoken largely in terms of largely black and white. In 2008 The American Medical Association (AMA) apologized for its past history of racial inequality toward African American physicians. This represents the first acknowledgment of a bitter truth: racism has pervaded medicine, as it has all aspects of American life. There are indeed important points to take away from this. The AMA, the parent organization of all local and state medical societies, was acutely aware of these discriminatory practices that were pervasive across the country and turned a blind eye to the actions and inactions of their organizational members.

By so doing, it tacitly endorsed discrimination, failing to represent the interests of African American physicians. The apology can be understood in the context social responsibility relevance that is morally and ethically relevant. There is also an acknowledgement in the AMA's apology of the scientific relevance of these discriminatory practices in medicine and their societal consequences that have contributed to the diminished health status of minority populations in the United States.

As early as 1906, W.E.B Du Bois wrote about the health disparities between blacks and whites in his report *The Health and Physique of the Negro American*. In 1914, Booker T. Washington, the founder of Tuskegee Institute, noted that the poor health of black Americans was an obstacle to economic progress. He called for "the negro people to join in a movement which shall be known as Health Improvement Week". As the years went by, the Negro Health Week evolved into a year round program known as the National Negro Health Movement. The movement was disbanded as America moved towards racial integration with the hope that blacks would be integrated and would benefit from the same programs as white Americans.

According to the most recent census, while African Americans, Hispanics, and Native Americans represent 27 percent of the United States population, they constitute less than 11 percent of nurses and 8 percent of physicians. The long history of racism continues to short change our national recruitment and retention of minority health care providers thus contributing to the racial and ethnic heath disparities.

The brutal treatment of the Native Americans is often not part of the discussion on racism in health care. A long history of treaties and broken promises is responsible for the dire situations that Native Americans face today. They are dying of alcoholism at a rate five times the national average, and they are facing rising numbers of tuberculosis, suicides, and diabetes. In the past ten years, there has been a 54 percent increase in newly diagnosed cases of suicide among teenage Native Americans. Although causes of and solutions to these problems have been identified by the Indian Health services (HIS), a branch of the U.S Department of Health and Human services, congress has not pushed forward any action plan. From a historical perspective, this should come as no surprise.

Today, the face of racism has become multi-colored and multicultural. With the influx of diverse populations entering the United States, racism has expanded to include antagonism between peoples of many cultures. A race is generally defined as a group of people with a common background. Race is a socially defined construct rather than a biological one. In the United States of America, race is categorized into: white, black, Latino or Hispanic, Asian, Pacific Islanders, and Native Americans. Ethnicity, however, adds a different dimension because it usually groups people by their common language and rituals.

Although they are different, race and ethnicity are used interchangeably and seen as one and the same especially in the busy life of the health care professional. A prominent visual cue in the first initial contact between the health professional and client can determine the care giver's interpretation of the client's race: the color of his or her skin. Many studies have shown that unfortunately the quality and accessibility of care are often determined on this factor regardless of a client's socioeconomic status, education level, and insurance coverage.

Racism, like our worst family secrets, is kept tightly wrapped and boxed in the closet. Schools and universities have their admission departments on alert to avoid any appearance of it. Hospitals openly tout their diversity programs and health care professionals proudly proclaim that they do not see color. Politicians denounce or embrace it to gain votes and many institutions will ensure that they publicize their equal opportunity policy to distance themselves from it. What lurks beneath all the rhetoric however can be easily brought to light if only our officials will take the time to look at current statistics. Numbers do not lie. The number of times a politician will resort to the race card, the number of minority managers in corporation, the number of minorities that succumb to medical errors, the number of minority candidates accepted into schools of nursing, the number of student nurses of color who are unable to pass beyond the first year of nursing programs, and the low quality care or negative outcomes because of the color blindness of some health care professionals.

Many will defend their color blindness as treating everyone the same. Everyone is not the same. Color- blind racism today enables individuals to perpetuate a covert ideological armor used to protect institutions. Those who assert that they do not see skin color must realize that it is not a compliment to the person of color. We want to be seen because we are not invisible or insignificant. Health care professionals need to realize that in twenty first century America, being color blind does not absolve them from the blemish of racism.

For a very brief period, the Institute of Medicine (IOM) report caused some ripples in the media when it was first published. The report firmly concluded that "although myriad sources contribute to these disparities, some evidence suggests bias, prejudice, and stereotyping on the part of health care providers may contribute to the differences in care". The IOM report, the Department of Health and Human Services, Healthy People 2000 and Healthy People 2010 have brought to the forefront the decades of health gaps that have prevailed "ever since accurate federal record keeping began". Still Americans either do not realize or willingly remain oblivious to this moral injustice. Researchers have substantiated that minorities receive a lower quality of care even though they carry the same insurance as their white counterparts. These findings are nothing new.

The disparity/inequality towards minorities, the poor, the elderly, and women does not seem to be newsworthy. It is not salacious enough to gain the public interest. Van Ryn and Burke (2000) even found in their research that white doctors often rated black patients as less intelligent, less educated, more likely to abuse drugs and alcohol, and less compliant. In this research, the findings remained constant even after patients' higher education and income status were taken into account. This clearly showed that health care providers' attitudes and perceptions are influenced by race.

Since 1787 there has been an agreement between the Federal government and Indian tribes that health care will be provided free of charge to those residing on the reservations through the Indian Health Service (IHS), a branch of the Department of Health and Human Services. Approximately 55 percent of American Indians (AI) and Alaska Natives (AN) rely on the IHS for their health care access. That sounds like a great deal, but despite the hundred of millions of dollars spent, the program is in crisis and reveals some significant disparities. The government allocates about fifty cents for every dollar needed by the IHS to provide just adequate services. Many of their clinics are not equipped to provide urgent care or handle serious conditions. The clinics must "buy" health care from larger medical facilities. The health money that Congress provides for the contract health care services is rarely sufficient, forcing many clinics to make "life or limb" decisions.

When it comes to health and disease in Indian country, the statistics are staggering. Those living outside of the reservation are often without insurance and unable to access necessary health care. American Indians have an infant death rate that is nearly twice the rate for whites. They are three times as likely to die from diabetes, 60 percent more likely to have a stroke. They are dying of alcoholism, tuberculosis, and suicide at an alarming rate. American Indians have disproportionately high death rates from unintentional injuries and a high prevalence of risk factors for obesity, substance abuse, sudden infant death syndrome, teenage pregnancy, liver disease and hepatitis.

The office of minority health at the U.S. Department of Health and Human Services, which oversees the Indian Health Service, notes on its Web site that American Indians "frequently contend with issues that prevent them from receiving quality medical care". These issues are as varied as the number of tribes. Social, cultural, structural, and financial barriers contribute to the health care disparities.

In 2006 Ta'Shon Rain Little Light, a happy little girl who loved to dance and dress up in traditional American Indian clothes, suddenly stopped eating and walking. She complained constantly to her mother that her stomach hurt. Stephanie Little Light took her daughter to the Indian Health Service clinic in this windswept and remote corner of Montana. She was told her the five year-old was depressed. Ta'Shon's pain rapidly worsened and over several months she visited the clinic about ten more times before her lung collapsed. She was then airlifted to a children's hospital in Denver. There she was diagnosed with terminal cancer and a few weeks later she died. Ta'Shon's story is not unique in the Indian Health Service system, which serves almost two million American Indians in thirty five states. This story has been well publicized, but did not cause much outraged.

A long history of broken treaties and mistrust compounded by lack of education, poverty, and poor housing are responsible for the dire situation. More than once, we have heard stories recounted by Senator Byron Dorgan, Democrat from North Dakota, of poor care that have produced disastrous outcomes. Dorgan's swath of the country is the hardest hit in terms of American Indian health care. Many of the reservations in North Dakota are poor, isolated, devoid of economic development opportunities and subject to long and harsh winters. Last year senator Dorgan persuaded Senate Majority Leader Harry Reid to consider an Indian health improvement bill that would have directed Congress to provide $35 billion for American Indian programs in the next ten years. The bill passed in the Senate. A similar bill died in the House after it became entangled in an abortion dispute. A few lawmakers in Washington have tried to bring attention to the broken system of health care for Native Americans as Congress attempts to improve health care for millions of other Americans.

The fastest growing minority group in America is the Hispanic population; however, a large portion of this population remains on the fringe of society and in the shadows. Hispanics are varied in culture, language, and socioeconomic status. The vast majority of Hispanics occupies the lower end of the income scale or lives below the poverty line. Even when employed, they are rarely offered health insurance through their employers. Research has shown that Hispanics are twice as likely as African Americans and three times as likely as non-Hispanic whites to lack access to health care. A recent Pew Hispanic Center study revealed that one out of four Hispanic Americans does not have a regular healthcare provider. In the past five years, those who have received health care report poor quality care and covert resentment due to language barriers, poverty, race/ethnicity, or stereotyping during the clinical encounters.

Researchers lament that many Hispanics do not come forward to complain about the quality of their care due to cultural norm or fear of jeopardizing their residential status. Recent research shows that obesity, diabetes and hypertension are reaching epidemic proportions. Poor nutrition, consuming excessive alcohol, smoking, and stress all contribute to the prevalence of negative outcomes on their health and wellness. Studies show that adult undocumented immigrants seldom use public health programs because of finances, mistrust and language barriers. Programs targeted toward children have higher rates of use.

In the past decade, the greatest gaps in life expectancy occur between Whites and African Americans. White females' life expectancy is 80 years compared to African American females whose life expectancy range around seventy- five years. The gap is greater for males. White males' life expectancy range around seventy-five but African American males' life expectancy is sixty-eight years. Deaths from diabetes are disproportionate in African American, Hispanic, and Native American populations ranging from five to ten times higher than the general population. Whites have an infant mortality rate of 6.7 percent compared to a rate of 12.5 percent for American Indians and 13.6 percent for

African Americans. Asthma, which is a leading cause of school absences, affects African American children twice as much as white children due to certain environmental factors. Roughly 4 percent of pre-school minority students have enough lead in their blood to reduce intelligence and attention span, causing learning disabilities. Over 90 percent of all lead poisoning cases in New York City involve children of color living in only ten neighborhoods known for their poor minority residents.

Many studies have shown that African American adults have a death rate from cardiovascular disease that is 30 percent higher than whites. Although African Americans and Hispanics comprise 25 percent of the population, they represent 55 percent of adult AIDS cases and 82 percent of pediatric AIDS cases. Given these statistics, how can we still think that the inequality of health care in the United States is not due to racism? Racism in medicine and racial biases of health care professionals in the United States must be acknowledged as contributing causes and risk factors for the current disparate health status and poor outcomes affecting blacks and populations of color.

The many issues of race and who bears the brunt of current prejudices and hatred are ever-shifting with the passing of time. Its burden and privileges shift like sand with the tide. The racial differences of the early days of Italians and Irish immigrants have now blended with the Caucasian majority to give rise to another facet of American immigration. Those coming to America in the twentieth and twenty first century are easily identifiable. They are very visible due to their skin color and their un-American accents. Even when they are better educated or of a higher socioeconomic status than their Caucasian counterparts, studies have found that they are subjected to many forms of overt and covert racism.

Hispanics are currently the largest minority group in the country and growing exponentially. They carry a disproportionately significant burden of diabetes and other chronic illnesses when compared to other segments of the population. It is in our best interests as a nation to address these disparities in a meaningful way. The lack of preventive health care for such a significant part of the population will eventually have a widespread economic impact on American society. According to a Pew Hispanic Center survey of Latino adults, eight in ten report receiving their health information from media sources or church groups. Countless studies have shown that people of color suffer higher rates of catastrophic illness and disease, and are much less likely to obtain basic drugs, tests, preventive screenings and surgeries.

Studies have found that when blacks and Hispanics do seek medical treatments, the care they receive is more likely to be substandard. In the past decade, there have been numerous reports showing that even when blacks and Hispanics are enrolled in high quality health plans, the care and quality of medical treatment are still substandard to that of their white counterparts. Although these undeniable statistics are currently available for all to read, many continue to debate whether race is the real issue. Poverty, language barrier, poor education, and even gender are some of the factors that collectively or individually have been attributed to health care disparities or inequities. To be fair to those debaters, each factor should be examined. *A Case for Closing the Gap* highlights some of the glaring disparities that exist in the current health system:

- 48 percent of all African Americans adults suffer from a chronic disease compared to 39 percent of the general population.
- 8 percent of white Americans develop diabetes while 15 percent of African Americans, 14 percent of Hispanics, and 18 percent of American Indians develop diabetes.
- Hispanics are one-third less likely to be counseled on obesity than are whites: only 44 percent of Hispanics received counseling.
- African Americans are 15 percent more likely to be obese than whites.

As mentioned earlier, eliminating disparities in health is part of the goals set forth in the Healthy People 2010 agenda. The disparities in the prevention, recognition, and treatment of cardiovascular disease among minorities are well documented from the many studies, articles, and books that have emerged in the past decade. Despite the equal disparity of care in all of the minority groups, the greatest focus has been on African American populations, with relatively little work related to Hispanic, Asian, Pacific Islanders, and Native American populations.

For decades, experts have agreed that racial disparities in health spring from pervasive social and institutional forces. The scientific literature has linked higher rates of death and disease in American blacks to such "social determinants" as residential segregation, environmental waste, joblessness, unsafe housing, targeted marketing of alcohol and cigarettes, and other inequities. Other researchers have suggested that racism acts as a classic chronic stressor, setting off the same physiological train wreck as job strain or marital conflict: higher blood pressure, elevated heart rate, and huge increases in the stress hormone Cortisol. Chronic stress is also known to encourage unhealthy behaviors, such as smoking and eating too much, thereby perpetuating the never ending cycle of risky behaviors and disease. Jules Harrell, a Howard University professor of psychology, said he was moved by a photo of the Rutgers University women's college basketball team sitting together with dignified expressions, after radio talk show host Don Imus had labeled them with a racist epithet. "The expressions on their faces" said Harrell. "All I could think was, 'Good God, I'd hate to see their cortisol levels' ".

A Harvard School of Public Health social epidemiologist Nancy Krieger pushed the hypothesis further. She confirmed that experiences of race-based discrimination were associated with higher blood pressure, and that an internalized response, not talking to others about the experience or not taking action against the inequity, will raise blood pressure even more. A controversial finding a decade ago, this finding has since been replicated by other investigators. The suppressed inner turmoil after a racist encounter can set off a cascade of ill effects.

Collectively, many studies of the racism-health link have tied experiences of discrimination to poorer self-reported health, smoking, low-birth-weight deliveries, depressive symptoms, and especially to cardiovascular effects. From laboratory work in the 1980 to real- life experiments, several investigations have linked blood pressure to real-time experiences of stress and discrimination as recorded in electronic diaries. In a 2008 study,

Elizabeth Brondolo, a psychologist at St. John's University, found that daytime experiences of racism led to elevated nighttime blood pressure, suggesting that the body could not turn off its stress response.

Despite these compelling findings, the field remains beset by unknowns. In the mid-1980s scientists began to take advantage of the controlled conditions of the laboratory. When African American volunteers were hooked up to blood-pressure monitors, for example, and then exposed to a racially provocative vignette on tape or TV -- such as a white store clerk calling a black customer a racial epithet -- the volunteers' blood pressures rose, their heart rates jumped, and they took longer than normal to recover from both reactions. Perhaps, scientists reasoned, the effort of a lifetime of bracing for such threats prolongs the effect.

One of the biggest problems is that researchers don't share a concrete, agreed-upon definition of racial discrimination partly because such prejudice takes myriad forms. They also don't know if more exposure to racism produces more disease or if, instead, disease sets in only after a threshold has been passed. They don't know if exposures during certain periods of life are more risky than others. And they don't know why some victims cope better than others.

In many studies, researchers have found unintentional racism, very often physicians are unaware of their biased feelings which affect how they diagnose and treat patients of color. A study by the Disparities Solutions Center, affiliated with Harvard University and Massachusetts General Hospital, was the first to deal with unconscious racial bias and how it can lead to inferior care for

African-American patients. The doctors in the study were told of two fictional male patients, one black and one white, each aged fifty with complaints and symptoms of chest pain. The result was most of the doctors were more likely to prescribe a potentially life-saving, clot-busting treatment for the white patients than for the African-American patient. Published in the online edition of the Journal of General Internal Medicine this study revealed that "physicians, like many others in the United States demonstrated unconscious biases based on race". According to the study, those biases affected the treatment doctors would have given the two patients.

Skeptics distrust people's own accounts of racial discrimination, because the experiences can't be objectively documented and because the victim can't always know the motives of the perpetrator. Racism and discrimination are social constructs of attitudes, beliefs, behaviors and practices that contribute to long- standing disparities in health. Racism affects health through a complicated set of direct physiologic effects, most notably physiologic stress, and through indirect pathways such as access to goods, services and opportunities. Analysis of such effects has proven difficult, in part because race and racism are difficult to quantify.

There is a common tendency in the United States that when dealing with the matter of racism, to limit the concept to individual random acts of prejudice (Feagin & McKinney, 2003). The nature of this phenomenon is so subtle and complex that experts in diversity training and cultural competence find it hard to unmask. It is so internalized and has permeated so many levels of the health care institutions that racism still determines the quality and quantity of care received by minority patients (Jones, 2000).

In 2009 secretary of U.S. Health and Human Services (HHS), Kathleen Sebelius, in June 2009 released a new report on health disparities in America. "Minorities and low income Americans are more likely to be sick and less likely to get the care they need" Secretary Sebelius said. "These disparities have plagued our health system and our country for too long. Now, it's time for Democrats and Republicans to come together to pass reforms this year that help reduce disparities and give all Americans the care they need and deserve".

Although the disparity in access to and quality of health care for minorities has fueled the crisis and the urgency for reform, the private insurers and hospitals will not openly state their biggest fear: required coverage to treat the millions of blacks and Hispanics who are uninsured. According to the Commonwealth Fund, nearly half of the estimated forty seven million Americans who have no health care insurance are in the minority groups, primarily because minority workers are mainly in low- paying jobs or work for companies that do not provide their workers health insurance. Since Harry Truman proposed the first national health care plan in the late 1940s, every Democratic president has had to wrestle with the overwhelming racial disparity in the number of uninsured. The massive public attention and anger over the health care crisis have caused insurers, their lobbyists and their political allies to find innovative ways to derail any reform. Although a few of the larger insurance companies have vowed their support for the current initiative, they are still scheming behind closed doors on how to exclude coverage to those labeled "high risk" or "undesirables."

Millions of minority patients who suffer chronic and major diseases—cancer, diabetes, asthma and heart disease- fall into the high risk category for health insurance. It is therefore imperative to eliminate the "pre-existing" clause in the reformed health care package. Blacks and Latinos have higher incidences of these ailments than whites, and they have been excluded from equal access to quality health care for years due to deeply held biases, entrenched institutional policies, and distrust. The battle for health care reform will again be a titanic struggle between a health care industry that has for decades resisted and successfully gutted every plan for expanded inclusive care. If individual illnesses are examined to compare access and quality of care, statistics will show that African Americans are twelve percent less likely to be recommended for coronary angioplasty and one-third less likely to receive bypass surgery than are whites. Heart disease and HIV/Aids are still showing the biggest discrepancies in term of recommended treatment. When compared to white patients, African Americans with HIV infection are less likely to be on antiretroviral therapy, less likely to receive prophylaxis for *pneumocystis* pneumonia, and less likely to receive protease inhibitors. With data showing such disparity in treatment, many researchers conclude that the great challenge is mainly minority recruitment during clinical trials.

The sad truth is that while only nine percent of African American patients are affected with AIDS, the mortality is three to four times higher than their white counterparts. Among preschool children hospitalized for asthma, only seven percent of black and two percent of Hispanic children, compared with twenty- one percent of white children, are prescribed routine medications to prevent future asthma-related hospitalizations. As for breast cancer studies and numerous data have shown that the length of time between an abnormal screening mammogram and the follow-up diagnostic test to determine whether a woman has breast cancer is more than twice as long in Asian American, black, and Hispanic women as in white women. Cancer statistics show that minority groups are more likely than the general population to develop and die from certain types of cancer. According to the Office of Minority Health in the Department of Health and Human Services:

- African Americans are more likely than any racial and ethnic group to die from all cancers combined and for most major cancers.
- American Indians/Alaska Natives are more likely than non-Hispanic whites to develop liver cancer.
- Asian Americans/Pacific Islanders are twice as likely as non-Hispanic whites to die from stomach cancer.
- Hispanics are more likely to develop cancers related to viral infection. For example, Hispanic women have the second highest number of cervical cancer cases. Cervical cancer is related to the human papillomavirus (HPV).

Minorities, due to a long history of suspicious treatment within the health care system, are very reluctant to participate in any research. Researchers and health care professionals insist that lack of research studies involving minorities is one of the barriers to early detection and screening. Language, cultural beliefs, and unequal access are among some of the reported barriers. In a new report cited by Reuters in May 2009, indicated that discrimination is rampant. Appropriate medications for a variety of diseases are often underprescribed, overprescribed, or misprescribed for African Americans, Hispanics and Asian Americans.

A comprehensive review of studies on medication use in U.S. minority groups, entitled "Origins and Strategies for Addressing Ethnic and Racial Disparities in Pharmaceutical Therapy: The Health-Care System, the Provider, and the Patient" clearly showed that disparities currently exist in the treatment of minority patients with cardiovascular illness, asthma, pain, psychiatric illness, and various other life- threatening conditions such as diabetes and renal failure. One case often made by health care professionals is that medication adherence in minority populations has been correlated with reduced adverse health outcomes. This argument diverts divert attention from the real problems that plaque the minority populations. Much of the association between race/ ethnicity and low medication adherence is due to low household income, lack of insurance, poor education, low health literacy, language barriers and cultural beliefs.

Language barriers exist for a broader group than just non-English speaking Americans. Health literacy applies to many Americans, especially the elderly. It includes extremely important concepts like the client's understanding of instructions on medication bottles, appointment slips, medical education brochures, consent forms, and their ability to negotiate complex issues within the health care system. Health literacy requires the client to read, listen, analyze, and make decision, and to apply these skills to understanding health situations. A person may have no problem functioning adequately at home or work but may be at a lost when dealing with the jargons and medical terminology in a health care environment. Efforts are underway to move toward a "consumer-centric" health care system in an effort to improve the quality of health care and to reduce unnecessary medical errors and health care costs.

In order to receive appropriate quality care, patients need to articulate their health concerns and describe their symptoms accurately. They need to ask pertinent questions, and they need to understand spoken medical advice or treatment directions. In an age of shared responsibility for health care between patients and physicians,, patients need strong decision-making skills. In *Health Literacy: A Prescription to End Confusion*, the Institute of Medicine reports that ninety million adults in the United States have difficulty understanding and using health information. Very often, simple instructions on how to take medications are misunderstood. Two- thirds of U.S. adults age sixty and over have inadequate or marginal literacy skills, and eight-one percent of patients age sixty and older at a public hospital could not read or understand basic materials like prescription labels. A large percentage of minority populations, immigrant populations, and low- income populations which amounts to approximately half of Medicare/Medicaid recipients read below the fifth-grade level.

According to the Agency for Health Care Research and Quality report, *Literacy and Health Outcomes* (January 2004), low health literacy is linked to higher rates of hospitalization and higher use of expensive emergency services. This evidence-based literature review highlighted numerous studies that provide a detailed analysis of the correlation between low health literacy and poor health. Patients with asthma, high blood pressure, and diabetes who are health illiterate can only read at a sixth- grade level or less. They have significantly less or no knowledge of their disease, important lifestyle modifications, and essential self-management skills. When in need of treatment, they reported that they use the emergency departments. There are economic consequences of low health literacy to society. Additional health care costs due to low health literacy are calculated at $125 billion dollars a year. Medicare pays about 35 percent of these expenditures and Medicaid pays more than $20 billion. Most of the additional expenditure is financed through FICA taxes on workers.

Hard working middle class Americans and the government are already paying large sums of money to sustain an inefficient system. There are many reasons why the system is inefficient, bleeding money, and catapulting toward bankruptcy. Medical costs have been rising faster than education, energy, and homeland security combined. National health spending is expected to reach $2.5 trillion in 2009. Many economists and health care experts estimate that up to 30 percent of health care is unnecessary, emphasizing the need to streamline the health system and eliminate needless spending. How can public payment programs like Medicare and Medicaid create market leadership toward desired change in the system, specifically as it relates to a fair reimbursement approach?

Over the last decade, employer-sponsored health insurance premiums have increased 119 percent. Employees have seen their share of job-based coverage increase at nearly the same rate during this period jumping from $1,545 to $3,354. And this year, many hospitals are rumored to be negotiating increased insurance cost and decreased coverage for their employees. In just three years, the Medicare and Medicaid programs will account for 50 percent of all national health spending. Indeed, the problem of medical costs is so pervasive that close attention is needed toward the increasingly rapid unraveling of employer-based health insurance.

Numerous failed attempts to introduce universal health insurance due to fearmongering and powerful lobbyists leave Americans with a system in which the government pays directly or indirectly for more than half of the nation's health care while private insurers, private hospitals, and other players increase consumers' costs without adding value. Americans have been so brain- washed into believing that curbing the cost of insurance companies will mean fewer options, care rationing, and the formation of "Death Panels" for the elderly that they cannot see logically and intelligently the true benefits of health care reform. Fear has always been the tactic used to deter hard- working Americans from choosing what would be of benefit to them instead of what would benefit those guarding their huge profits. We could do even better if we learned from "integrated" systems such as the Veterans Administration that directly provide some health care as well as medical insurance.

Costs have emerged as a central element of any national health reform effort. As policymakers move forward with plans to enact comprehensive health reform, costs will surely continue to be at the forefront of the surrounding policy debates. Arguments to retain the status quo will be the same refrain: cost, inefficiency, heavy-handed government control and interference. The furor will intensify if there is any mention of race. Conservative talk show hosts and commentators will demonize anyone trying to have open discussions on this very important issue. They will as always try to muddy the waters by throwing into the mix the idea of socialism, government take over, and health care for illegal immigrants. More control and power to the insurance companies will be briefly discussed by some news anchors while some key players in government will try to negotiate plans that strive to maintain the enormous profit margins of the insurance and pharmaceutical companies. Inequities and disparities might be mentioned briefly. Race, of course, will be totally omitted from the conversation.

University of Dayton School of Law Professor, Vernellia Randall, outlines nine factors through which the race paradigm affects healthcare training and delivery systems: (1) lack of economic access to health care; (2) barriers to hospitals and healthcare institutions; (3) barriers to physicians and other providers; (4) discriminatory policies and practices; (5) lack of language and culturally-competent care; (6) inadequate inclusion in healthcare research; (7) commercialization of healthcare; (8) disintegration of traditional medicine; and (9) disparities in medical treatment.

Over a century ago, the great W. E. B. DuBois noted racial and ethnic disparities. At the time, he posited that health disparities revealed a "vast set of problems having a common center that must be studied according to a general plan." In many surveys done in the past five years, doctors stated that treatment can be further equalized with universal insurance coverage, more data on race, more awareness of disparities, and medical improvements like linking doctor and hospital payments to performance. These recommendations have been tried and implemented by some with great success, but obviously more must be done to reverse the trends.

In 2005, Congress passed a bill that required everyone applying for Medicaid to show documentation proving that they were citizens. In the confusion that ensued, Congress discovered that not many illegal immigrants were trying get enroll. The huge bureaucratic nightmare was not with people here illegally getting on Medicaid. In fact, those who are illegal tend to avoid coming forward and interacting with government programs mostly for fear of getting caught. However, a lot of people who were citizens and eligible for Medicaid were being locked out of the system. Many of the legal citizens, the elderly, the poor, and those most in need were not able to come up with the required documents, either their birth certificates or actual copies of hospital papers or drivers' licenses. Many of those who need to apply do not possess drivers' licenses or passports. People who are eligible for Medicaid do not tend to travel to other countries. Among those being denied were a large number of Native Americans who failed to produce the required documents that they were actually citizens of the United States. Did this make the news cycle? Was it repeated, analyzed, and discussed by the so called experts? These racial issues are rarely discussed openly in our society.

When listening to many of our conservative politicians, one would assume that it is very easy for the underinsured and the uninsured to access health care within an extensive safety net of health care facilities, emergency departments, outpatient clinics, and nonprofit community hospitals. This somehow absolves their guilt and excuses their paternalistic attitudes. But for those privileged individuals do not know how difficult it is for the underprivileged to access health care. They have never been in that predicament.

I will end this chapter by bringing to light the vitriol heard concerning health care coverage for illegal immigrants. When conservatives discuss illegal immigrants these days, they are really referring to Hispanics, Latino, Chicano- anyone originating from South or Central America. The arguments from the right are all about making sure that these brown invaders do not receive any care if they are sick.

REFERENCES:

Adler N. E, & Newman K. (2002). Socioeconomic disparities in health: Pathways and policies. *Health Affairs* 21(2):60-76.

Bayne-Smith, M. (1996). Health *and Women of Color: Race, gender, and health.* Thousand Oaks, CA: Sage.

Bhopal, R. (1998). Spectre of racism in health and health care: Lessons from history and the United States. *British Medical Journal,* 316: 1970-1973.

Brondolo, E., Rieppi, R., Kelly, K. P., & Gerrin W. (2003). Perceived racism and blood pressure: A review of the literature and conceptual and methodological critique. *Ann Behav Med. 25:* 55-65.

Brown ER, Ojeda VD, Wyn R, Levan R. (2000). *Racial and Ethnic Disparities in Access to Health Insurance and Health Care.* Los Angeles, CA: UCLA Center for Health Policy Research and the Henry J. Kaiser Family Foundation.

Byrd W. M, & Clayton L.A. (2002). *An American Health Dilemma: Race, Medicine, and Health Care in the United States 1900-2000,* Vol. 2. New York: Routledge

Cohen, H. & Northridge, M. (2000). Getting Political: Racism and urban health. *American Journal of Public Health, Vol. 90*: 841-842.

Collins K.S, Tenney K, & Hughes D.L. (2002). *Quality of health care for African Americans: Findings from the Commonwealth Fund 2001 Health Care Quality Survey.* New York: The Commonwealth Fund.

Du Bois, W.E.B. (1906). *The Health and Physique of the Negro American.* Atlanta, GA: Atlanta University Press.

Freeman H., & Payne, R. (2000). Racial Injustice in Health Care. *N. England Journal Med.342*: 1045-1047.

Galanti, G. (1997). *Caring for Patients of Different Cultures.* Philadelphia: University of Pennsylvania Press.

Gamble, V. N. (1997). Under the Shadow of Tuskegee: African American and Health care. *American Journal of Public Health, 87(11)*: 1773--1778

Geiger J. 2003. *Unequal Treatment: Confronting Racial and Ethnic Disparities in Health Care.* Institute of Medicine. Smedley BD, Stith AY, Nelson AR, eds. Washington, DC: The National Academies Press.

Karlsen, S. & Nazroo, J.Y. (2002).Agency and Structure: The impact of ethnic identity and racism on the ethnic minority people. *Sociol Health Illness, 24:* 1-20.

Korenbrot CC, Ehlers S, Crouch JA. 2003. Disparities in hospitalizations of rural American Indians. *Medical Care* 41(5):626-636.

National Center for Health Statistics, United States, 2004. With Chartbook on trends in the Health of Americans. Hyattsville, MD: National Center for Health Statistics.

Physicians for Human Rights (PHR). (2003). *The Right to Equal Treatment: An Action Plan to End Racial and Ethnic Disparities in Clinical Diagnosis and Treatment in the United States.* [Organizational Report]. Boston, MA: Author.

Savitt, T. L. (1982). The Use of Blacks for Medical experimentation and Demonstration in the Old South. *Journal of Southern History, 48*: 331-348.

Stone, J. (2002). Race and Health Care Disparities Overcoming Vulnerability. *Theoretical Medicine, 23*: 499—518.

U.S Department of Health and Human Services (2001). *Healthy People 2010. Understanding and Improving Health.* Boston: Jones and Bartlett Publishers.

U.S Department of Health and Human Services, Office of Minority Health, Public Health Services. CDC awards funding to community for projects to help eliminate racial and ethnic disparities. [Press release] September 30, 1999, Washington DC.

van Ryn M. 2002. Research on the provider contribution to race/ethnicity disparities in medical care. *Medical Care* 40(1):I140-I151.

van Ryn M, Burke J. 2000. The effect of patient race and socio-economic status on physician's perceptions of patients. *Social Science and Medicine* 50:813-828.

Washington, B.T. Quoted by Patterson F. Statement concerning National Negro Health Week. *Negro Health News,* 1939, 7: 13.

Williams D.R., Yu, Y., Jackson, J.S., & Anderson N.B. (1997). Racial differences in physical and mental health: Socio-economic status, stress, and discrimination. *Journal of Health Psychol.* 2: 335-351.

Williams, D.R., & Rucker, T.D. (2000). Understanding and addressing racial disparities in health care. *Minority Health,* 2(1): 30-39.

*Health is the greatest gift, contentment the greatest wealth, faithfulness
the best relationship.*

Buddha *(563 BC-483 BC)*
founder of Buddhism.

CHAPTER 2
GENDER AND POVERTY

Until a decade ago, medical research, including drug studies frequently excluded women. There was a long-standing belief that men and women "were biologically the same except for their reproductive organs" said Sherry Marts of the Society for Women's Health Research. The National Women's Law Center, an advocacy group that has examined hundreds of individual insurance policies, found that women - both young and middle aged - pay dramatically more in most states for individual health insurance than men.

Some major insurance companies offered many excuses for discriminating against women. In an article published by the New York Times, a senior vice president of Humana, Thomas Noland Jr. explained "Premiums for our individual health insurance plans reflect claims experience based on the use of medical services which varies by gender and age. Females use more medical services than males, and this difference is most pronounced in young adults." Noland went on to say, "Bearing children increases other health risks later in life, such as urinary incontinence, which may require treatment with medication or surgery." This claim is astonishing and although published in the New York Times, it was not seen as worthy news elsewhere.

Some insurance executives expressed surprise at the size and prevalence of the disparities, which can make a woman's insurance cost hundreds of dollars a year more than a man's. Women's advocacy groups have raised concerns about the differences, and members of Congress have briefly questioned the justification for them. In general, insurers say, they charge women more than men of the same age because claims experience shows that women use more health care services. They are more likely to visit doctors, to get regular checkups, to take prescription medications and to have certain chronic illnesses.

Marcia D. Greenberger, co-president of the National Women's Law Center said "The wide variation in premiums could not possibly be justified by actuarial principles. We should not tolerate women having to pay more for health insurance, just as we do not tolerate the practice of using race as a factor in setting rates."

Siminoff, Graham and Gordon (2006) studied oncologists and their female patients. One of the fascinating and disturbing findings was that oncologists tend to communicate differently with women newly diagnosed with breast cancer, depending on race, education, age and income. Visits between 58 oncologists and 405 women were videotaped and showed that the physicians spent more time engaged in building relationships with white women than with women of other races. The same was true of visits with more educated and affluent patients compared with less advantaged patients.

In keeping with their professional codes of ethics, health care providers must seize every opportunity to take a stand and to speak out against racism in health care in whatever form it assumes. To remain silent on this issue would be an abdication of professional moral responsibility. Silence could also be seen by others as giving assent and credence to racism in health care and thereby condoning (if not encouraging) the burden of suffering it imposes on people whose race and ethnicity others simply do not like. Researchers have identified a number of key processes commonly contributing to racial and ethnic disparities in health and quality care among minority groups. They include inadequate communication (relating to the lack of appropriate access to health interpreting services); the lack of a systematic (and national) approach to the culturally competent delivery of care to culturally and linguistically diverse populations; and the poor attitudes and disrespectful behaviors of some staff.

Less well acknowledged, however, is the degree to which individual and institutional racism have contributed to the status quo and which, unless recognized, cannot and will not be reconciled. Rarely expressed openly, racism can come in many guises (Levine & Pataki 2004). Racial and ethnic disparities in health and health care are just some of the many guises that racism can assume and stand as potent examples of just how insidious racism can be. After researching a wide range of data sources from federal agencies and other research organizations, Levine and Pataki showed that minority women continue to fare worse than white women in terms of health status, rates of disability, and mortality. Life expectancy for women of all races has nearly doubled over the past one hundred years, from 48 in 1900 to 79.5 in 2000, yet minority women continue to lag about five years behind white women. For example, in the most recent statistics, white women could expect to live to age 80 compared with 74.9 for black women.

The status of women in every state and the District of Columbia reflects a magnitude of disparities and inequities. Very often, health and patterns of health care are influenced by numerous factors beyond to health coverage. Personal behaviors such as smoking, diet and nutrition, early life experiences, psychosocial development, work environment, neighborhoods, and housing have a direct or indirect influence on health outcomes. One of the greatest social determinants of health and health care use is socioeconomic status, or social class, which is often measured by income, education, and occupation.

Women are more likely to live in poverty than men, and women of color are more likely than either white men or white women to live below the poverty line. These differences are often due to the fact that women are the head of single parent households and shoulder the major responsibility for raising children. The link between income and health is well established. Poor individuals are less likely to have access to health insurance, and less likely to have routine screenings and checkups.

Lack of access is associated with a higher risk of delays in care and potentially poorer health outcomes. Breast cancer screening is less common in counties that have many uninsured women. Routine mammography is a critical factor in helping to diagnose breast cancer in its earliest stages, when treatment is most effective. Minority women, especially African Americans, have a lower incidence of breast cancer but poorer survival rates when diagnosed. Many health care professionals believe that the cancer is detected when it is more advanced and more difficult to treat.

Poverty also indirectly affects health through factors like nutrition and stress. Women of color live in poverty at more than twice the rate of white women. Of all groups, American Indian and Alaska Native women experienced the highest poverty rates at 33 percent compared to 29 percent of black women, 27.8 percent of Hispanic women, and 12 percent of white women.

Over fifteen million households are headed by single parents, and the overwhelming majority are headed by single women. Households headed by single women are more likely to be poor, which affects the physical, psychological, and educational outcomes of the children raised in such an environment. Parents with limited economic resources face many obstacles to healthy living. Single mothers often report higher levels of psychological distress, lower levels of perceived social support, no insurance, and poorer eating habits. Those from racial and ethnic minority groups are more likely than whites to live in socioeconomically disadvantaged neighborhoods and such neighborhoods often have reduced access to public resources and healthy food, fewer employment opportunities, and greater exposure to hazardous health conditions.

Many researchers have posited that socioeconomic and racial segregation of neighborhoods can have strong effects on both neighborhood conditions and the health of residents. In medically underserved communities, primary care is therefore an essential component of the health care delivery system. With lack of access to primary care health providers, poor patients often visit the emergency departments of hospitals clogging the system and increasing costs. Almost half of women nationwide lived in an area where there is a shortage of primary care providers. More than four in ten women nationwide lived in an area with a shortage of mental health providers.

According to several indicators, American Indian and Alaska Native women have higher rates of health and access challenges than women in other racial and ethnic groups on several indicators, and often three to five times higher than the rates for whites. American Indian and Alaska Native women have higher rates of obesity, diabetes, and smoking. This pattern is generally evident throughout the country. One third of American Indian and Alaska Native women are uninsured or have not had any recent dental checkup or mammogram and are not getting early prenatal care. Latina women are also disproportionately poor with low educational status, factors that contribute to their overall health and access to care. Because many Hispanic women are immigrants, they do not qualify for publicly funded insurance programs like Medicaid even if they are here legally, and language barriers often make access and health literacy a greater challenge.

Among black women, the most striking disparity is the extremely high rate of new AIDS cases. The AIDS epidemic is strongly concentrated among women of color, particularly black women. While all women regardless of age, race, or socioeconomic status are affected by AIDS, this burden has fallen heaviest on black women. The epidemic has also had a disproportionate effect on Latinas and American Indian and Alaska Native women. Lack of economic and political power is believed to be a major factor contributing to the inequitable social and economic conditions that lead to the escalation of HIV disease among women of color. Policies that support HIV/AIDS prevention and treatment programs for women are greatly needed to reduce this disparity. A Centers for Disease Control study of more than twenty thousand patients with HIV in ten U.S cities reported that women were slightly less likely than men to receive prescriptions for the most effective treatments for HIV infection.

High- risk heterosexual contact is responsible for infecting most women with HIV. The dynamics that exist in these relationships play an important role. Lower education, lack of awareness of the risk factors, substance abuse, domestic violence, and lack of empowerment are among the factors that endanger many women, and those of color in disproportionate numbers. Black and Hispanic women account for over 85 percent of the women living with HIV/AIDS who acquired HIV through high-risk heterosexual contact. Many women cannot insist on condom use because of sexual inequality and the fear that their partner will physically abuse or leave them. The presence of some sexually transmitted diseases greatly increases the likelihood of acquiring or transmitting HIV infection. The rates of gonorrhea and syphilis are higher among women of color than among white women.

To take a serious look at the inequalities that plaque women's health, real discussions about education, poverty, and socioeconomic status as barriers to access and quality of care need to happen. Gender- based discrimination has always been part of health care, but the fact that the inequalities and disparities that exist within this group subjugate certain racial or ethnic groups more than others have never been openly discussed. The race factor still remains the elephant in the room. As report by the Institute of Medicine IOM, "The medical enterprise, both in scientific research and clinical practice, has traditionally viewed female lives and bodies through a lens of masculine experience and assumptions." Are we to continue to make these assumptions?

Health care reform cannot be truly successful unless all these inequalities are identified. Discussions about race always provoke such irrational behaviors. As posited by W. E. B Du Bois at the beginning of the twentieth century, "The problem of the twentieth century is the problem of the color line." Well into the twentieth century, race relations in America are still not equal despite all the laws and policies. Once again attention must be paid to institutional racism.

Most of the worst neighborhood, the worst schools, the highest rate of poverty and crime, and the highest unemployment levels in this country retain the distinction of ethnic ownership. Although the majority of Americans seem to be in favor of frank discussions on race, there is a profound backlash whenever anyone attempt to do so. U. S Attorney General Eric holder was rebuked when he voiced such an opinion. There was such an uproar over his candor. Pundits and the news media repeatedly claimed the notion that liberals are provoking racial tensions and playing the race card. And somewhere from the wilderness of the GOP two or three rare specimens of ethnic conservatives are shuffled from network to network to persuade viewers about the validity of their false choices and the path of destruction that the liberals have mapped for America through government takeover. There is such an aversion to balanced and intelligent conversation on race that any attempt is vilified and promptly locked in the closet for fear of revealing its true nature.

The privileged class always reverts to the fear tactics of socialism and government takeover in discussions of health care reform. Health care is considered a privilege by those who have it, and they pay handsomely for that privilege. Present health reform is being derailed partly by a well-financed disinformation campaign by groups currently known like Freedom Works, a registered non-profit that is heavily funded by undisclosed for-profit corporations. Before this group was re-branded with a fancy new name, it was known in the Clinton era as Citizens for a Sound Economy. What a grand name! You would be mistaken however to think that its focus is on the economic concerns of every citizen. Its concern is mainly safeguarding the bottom line of large corporations and defeating any initiative that would cut their profit margin. Protecting the welfare of the privileged and keeping the status quo alive are their primary goals. To achieve success, they need to recruit the help of those in the corridors of power and especially those who were sent to Congress by the American people.

With privilege and insider clout come the revolving door opportunities to pocket millions of dollars. About fifteen years ago one of the most ardent opponents of health care reform under President Clinton was Dick Armey. His needy constituents who elected him had faith that their best interests were his priorities. In retrospect, considering his involvements with FreedomWorks and opposition to the real equality of care for working and middle class Americans, millions of dollars in campaign contributions spoke louder than the real need of those who elected him.

Today, nothing much has changed. Prominent congressmen, some holding highly influential positions on major committees, are still being swayed by the millions of dollars of contributions to their campaigns from the very companies that need to be reformed. Corporate communism is the practice of the day... monopoly for the insurance industry and denial of choice and fair play for the American people. The insurance companies do not want to compete in a fair market. They want to keep a stranglehold on the health care industry. They are not ready to allow the less privileged Americans to have a shot at equitable health care. Regardless of reconciliations and negotiations that remain to be hammered out, many in Congress see no need for any reform and intend to crush it at the expense of not just the forty seven millions uninsured, but of those who are one illness away from a shattered life. But that is not the concern of the privileged...because to them health care is not a right but a privilege for those who can afford it!

REFERENCE

Aday, L.A. (2001). At risk in America: The health and health care needs of vulnerable populations in the United States (2nd. Ed). Jossey-Bass series.

American Cancer Society. *Cancer Facts & Figures 2005*. Atlanta: American Cancer Society; Available at:http://www.cancer. org/downloads/STT/CAFF2005f4PWSecured.pdf

American Heart Association. *Heart Disease and Stroke Statistics—2003 Update*. Dallas, TX: American Heart Association; 2002.

Arias E, Anderson RN, Kung HC, Murphy SL, Kochanek KD. Deaths: final data for 2001. *Natl Vital Stat Rep* 2003 Sep 18;52(3):1-115.

Freeman H, Aiken LH, Blendon RJ, Corey CR. Uninsured working-age adults: characteristics and consequences. *Health Serv Res* 1990 Feb;24(6):811-23.

Hadley J. *Sicker and Poorer: The Consequences of Being Uninsured*. The Kaiser Commission on Medicaid and the Uninsured; May 2002. (Executive Summary updated February 2003). Available at: www.kff.org/uninsured/20020510-index.cfm. Accessed April 13, 2005.

Mitchell S, Schlesinger M; AcademyHealth. (2004). Gender Disparities in Healthcare Experiences: The Impact of Managed Care Practices. *Abstr AcademyHealth Meet.* 2004; 21: abstract no. 1510.

Salganicoff A, Beckerman JZ, Wyn R, Ojeda VD. *Women's Health in the United States: Health Coverage and Access to Care*. Menlo Park, CA: Kaiser Family Foundation. 2002. Available at: www.kff.org/womenshealth/20020507a-index.cfm.

Smedley, B. (206). The state of Black America.: race, poverty, and health care disparities. *National Urban League*

Stone, k. Health care, Poverty, and Race. Retrieved from http:// www.fleshandstone.net/policy_trends/healthcareandrace. html.

Wilken, M., & Furlong, B. (2002). *Poverty and Health Care Disparities: Lessons and solutions for health care providers.* Emerald Group Publishing Ltd.

Williams, R. A. (2007). *Eliminating Healthcare Disparities in America: Beyond the IOM Report.* Humana Press Inc. NJ.

I was told by my "trusted" high school counselor that there was no such thing as a Black woman doctor; despite my being a member of the National Honor Society, President of my high school class, and a national YWCA youth leader. I was told that I should choose a profession more suited to my race.

Kimberlydawn Wisdom, M.D,
Michigan Surgeon General.

CHAPTER 3
INSTITUTIONAL RACISM
AND CULTURAL
COMPETENCE

In this chapter, consideration of institutional racism moves beyond beliefs and behaviors to the deeply ingrained structural and systemic factors and policies that affect an individuals' health. Institutional policies affect health care and thus health status through three main areas: access to care, the quality of care that is provided, and the scope and relevance of the care rendered. Organizational policies and attitudes that bring about different levels of access and quality of service to different populations, or that assume that all clients have the same range of needs, are major contributors to persistent health disparities. For instance, housing location and environmental quality are acknowledged to have an impact on health status yet they are rarely addressed in public health programs. Activities like cultural competence training that improve linguistic and cultural access to care have been researched and proven to be paramount in the health status of a culturally diverse population.

According to the 2002 Census, more than 31 percent of the population consists of ethnic minorities. Ethnic minorities are very interested in sustaining their identity, values, and belief system and want to be recognized in a bicultural, pluralistic, and multicultural manner (Bucher, 2000). By 2020, the population of ethnic minorities will increase to approximately 50 percent of the entire U.S. population (U.S. Department of Health and Human Services [DHHS], 2001). To respond to this demographic change in the United States, health care professionals must embrace the challenge of providing culturally competent care and be taught cultural competence. To enable the delivery of such care, all health care professionals but especially nurses, who are often the frontline care givers, need to be taught cultural competence. Cultural competence is the "process in which the health care professional continuously strives to achieve the ability and availability to effectively work within the cultural context of a client (individual, family, community)" (Campinha-Bacote, 2003, p. 23).

In the next few pages, I will focus mainly on the need to educate nursing students for the complex and demanding roles of taking care of a rapidly changing demographics. To face such complexities and challenges, nursing students need to be given the appropriate knowledge as soon as they start being student nurses. The dilemma for many existing nursing programs is the lack of expert faculty to teach culturally competent care (Ryan, Carlton, & Ali, 2000). As the client base becomes increasingly multicultural, nursing faculty remain predominantly Caucasian, middle-class women who have been immersed in the Anglo-Saxon way of interacting and teaching with the knowledge and belief of a predominantly Western caring system. Nursing and nursing education have traditionally been very Eurocentric, with a strong emphasis on individualism, time-orientation, linearity, and independence (Crow, 1993). Learning to value ethnic diversity involves appreciating how variations in culture and background may affect health care and acknowledging and responding to an individual's culture in its broadest sense, which requires health-care professionals to learn the skills to negotiate effective communication, to have a heightened awareness of one's own attitudes, and to have a sensitivity to issues of stereotyping, prejudice, and racism.

A culturally competent nurse is critically important for the success of not just the nursing profession, but for positive health outcomes of our patients. The primary goal of the health care professionals is to improve quality of care and to eliminate disparities. Imparting general knowledge about cultural concepts is not the best way to teach nursing students. The danger of stereotypes lies in generalities. Nurses should learn the critical elements of respect for the inherent rights of all our patients regardless of race, gender, age, or disability. Before they care for patients of diverse backgrounds, they need to acknowledge biases, personal beliefs, and differing lifestyles.

To keep abreast of patients' changing demographics and the need to reduce health disparities among minorities due to miscommunication, misunderstandings, or simply a lack of knowledge, the nursing profession needs clinicians who are aware, skillful, and proficient in working with clients of different cultures. The nation's population demographic outlook for the next century shows the numbers of minorities increasing, and health care issues will remain at the forefront of concerns for those growing populations. Under careful scrutiny, in the majority of hospitals and schools of nursing, when we look at nursing leaders, hospital CEOs, board members, faculty, and deans, we do not see a diverse picture. The mosaic is monochrome for the most part. It is therefore imperative for the health care system to focus on racially, culturally, and economically diverse populations in efforts to improve the distribution and retention of the nation's healthcare workforce. A draft of *Healthy People 2010: National Health Promotion and Disease Prevention Objectives*, by the U.S Department of Health and Human Services, stated, "Increasing the number of minority health professionals is viewed as a partial solution to improving access to care. Several studies have shown that underrepresented minority health profession graduates are more likely to enter primary care specialties and to voluntarily practice in or near designated primary care health workforce shortage areas."

When working with Latino families, health care professionals must consider the critical cultural factors of *respecto, familialism,* and prescribed gender roles are critical to consider. *Respecto* or respect dictates the appropriate differential behavior toward others on the basis of age, socioeconomic status, gender, and authority position. The concept of *familialism* determines reciprocal relationships of responsibility, loyalty, and support among family and extended family members. Most importantly, within Latino culture, there is a traditional prescription of roles that is based on gender. Nurses, who very often are the first to assess the patients and interact with the families, need to be very aware of the hierarchy and show respect for cultural values and practices held by their patients and their families.

Although health care professionals interpret the term cultural competence to mean awareness of the differences and respecting them, it is an integration of knowledge, attitudes, and skills needed to work with a very diverse clientele. In health care today, practitioners need to understand that even within one culture, values vary along a continuum. Inherent in any care giver-client interaction is communication. This process is sometimes fraught with pitfalls. When communicating with someone from a very different cultural background, which can be compounded by the fact that English is often the second language, the likelihood of miscommunication increases significantly. In many cultures, the person making the health- related decisions might not be the patient, and privacy of information is not determined on the same value system. To avoid needless complications, the boundaries must be explored and determined before mistakes are made.

The plight and experiences of the Hispanic population in the United States are of great concern and need to be understood by all health care providers. In addition, language barriers, poor housing conditions, low wages, and limited education opportunities are contemporary factors that influence health and well being. The practice of caring is just not the doing of what is expected by the organization in a day's work, but constitutes the complete involvement of the nurse as the patient's advocate and a total interactive agent.

For health care professionals to develop an understanding of diversity, they must understand their own "hot buttons" and discover how and perhaps why we they behave the way they we do. People respond to the behavior of those around them, not their intentions. Regardless of personal values, it is paramount that co-workers treat each other with respect and integrity. It is crucial that all health care professionals differentiate between stereotypes and generalizations.

Both the patient and the health care professional must be aware that senses of spatial distance are significant in cross cultural communication. For example, patients and families of Hispanic and Middle-Eastern origins might want to bring the health care professional more closely into their circle as a sign of comfort and respect, which might be perceived by the practitioner as an invasion of their personal space. This discomfort can be perplexing for the families, and the health care practitioner may be viewed as aloof and unfriendly. American, Canadian, and British people need more personal space whereas people from Latin America and the Middle East need the least. There are usually five types of nonverbal behaviors that convey information to the client: tone of voice, facial expressions, use of personal and territorial space, and touch. Wide cultural variations exist when interpreting silence and eye contact.

Violating norms related to appropriate male-female relationships may jeopardize the health care professional's therapeutic relationship with patients and their families. In many cultures, but especially among people from the Middle East, unrelated persons of the opposite sex cannot be left alone in closed proximity. Even a simple encounter of shaking hands while greeting might be found disrespectful and inappropriate. Especially for clients who have recently immigrated, and are in various stages of assimilation and acculturation, traditional customs are still very relevant. Nonverbal behaviors are culturally very significant, and failure to adhere to the *cultural code* is viewed as a serious transgression. The best way to know if the cultural variables are correct is to ask. It is better to establish a relationship of trust and respect very early on in the encounter.

According to Title VI of the Civil Rights Act of 1964, "No person in the United States shall, on ground of race, color, or national origin, be excluded from participation in, be denied the benefits of, or be subjected to discrimination under any program or activity receiving federal financial assistance." Many strategies and initiatives have been implemented to ensure that patients are not discriminated against. But very often attitudes get in the way. The Emergency Medical Treatment and Active Labor Act (EMTALA) is known by most physicians and emergency department staff as the Patient Anti-Dumping Statute. It requires hospitals that participate in the Medicare program to treat all patients (including women in labor) in an emergency without regard to their ability to pay. Hospitals that fail to provide language assistance to persons of limited English proficiency are potentially liable to federal authorities for civil penalties as well as relief to the extent deemed appropriate by a court. These are powerful safety nets that are in place to ensure that minorities and the poor are treated with dignity in their most vulnerable moments. Nevertheless, stereotyping and generalizations still get in the way of culturally congruent care. Stereotypes and generalizations are often very easy to resort to in a hectic health care environment. During encounters with culturally diverse patients different from their own cultural group, health care practitioners attribute a defined set of characteristics to a group of patients. Although it may be done with good intentions, labeling all Africans or South Americans or Asians as having the same values and beliefs can be negative. Minorities are disturbed by the perception of stereotyping and are threatened by the possibility of unfair treatment due to the generalization.

Language often is cited as a barrier to health care. Nearly thirty five millions people in the United States speak a language other than English. Physicians will inevitably treat people with limited or no English proficiency. Both law (Title VI of the Civil Rights Act of 1964) and good medicine require physicians to make the best attempt to communicate with these patients. Furthermore, the federal government requires any health care provider who receives federal funding from the Department of Health and Human Services to communicate with patients effectively or risk being sued when errors are made due to miscommunication.

There are several strategies for working through a language barrier. Becoming a bilingual provider should be the main goal, especially if medical students plan to work in an environment with a large population of non-English- speaking patients. Language banks are part of an unreliable system that uses the bilingual skills of unofficial volunteer interpreters. Although they are sometimes the only option, language banks are fraught with many problems, including time strain on the volunteer's "real" duties. Unlike official interpreters, hospital and clinic employees who volunteer at language banks tend to be untrained and therefore may incorporate bias into their interpretations. Ideally, a professional medical interpreter is the best choice. Medical interpreters can take on a variety of roles, depending on the needs of the provider and the patient. In situations where there may be cultural misunderstandings, a knowledgeable interpreter can be a valuable "culture broker" someone who knows about the cultures of both provider and patient and explains when cultural differences that may cause confusion. It is up to the provider, patient and interpreter to determine what kind of interpreter is needed. Ultimately, the provider should always watch the interaction between the interpreter and the patient.

Though the expense of professional interpreters is often cited as an obstacle, organizations should think of the more expensive monetary and ethical consequences. Poor communication can lead to worse health or liability costs. A provider in Washington, D.C., was sued for $11 million when, due to miscommunication, an abortion was performed on a non-English speaking woman who only wanted contraception. Another issue to be aware of is the use of family members, especially children, as interpreters. Not only is this role stressful for a child, but adult patients may lie or be reluctant to talk about sexual concerns or life-threatening illnesses when speaking through a child. Family members, similar to untrained interpreters, may incorporate bias into their interpretations. Also, there may be a disruption of family dynamics when children are consulted for their adult family member's medical problems.

Finally, community members and traditional healers such as shamans, *curanderos* and herbalists may be used to act as cultural brokers and interpreters. They are aware of the cultural differences between provider and patient and most believe in Western medicine in conjunction with traditional methods. Also, patients are more likely to stick with a treatment plan that incorporates their beliefs.

Creating multicultural organizations requires change at both the organizational level and the individual level. Organizations can change policies and the way they do business. Individuals can change behaviors that will allow the policies and mandates to work. All employees should strive to create an inclusive environment. For such a cultural change to be successful, fair and equitable practices must be in place from recruitment to retention. "Undoing" institutional racism is not one specific action, nor does it take place all at once. Organizational change has been defined as having four basic levels:

- Awareness: institutional definition and official acceptance of a problem
- Adoption: institutional willingness to address the problem

- Implementation: provision of resources and engagement
- Institutionalization: including evaluation and re-planning (an ongoing Process).

Although all four levels are critical components of successful change, the scope of change is determined in the awareness and adoption phases. One of the most important criteria for success is the willingness of the institution to take responsibility and implement real change. Conservative health policy thinkers and conservative voters in general deeply believe in personal responsibility for health and wellness. Claims of racial inequity in health and medical care are anathema because they tend to point blame away from patients and toward doctors, hospitals, health plans, the insurance companies, and the government. Conservatives frown upon talk of racial disparity in health care and discussions on public or private sector initiatives to reduce it. They believe that such ideas discourage citizens from taking care of themselves and promote the notion of big government take over. As President George W. Bush said, "Better health is an individual responsibility."

This is all well and good if you have the access, the resources, the comprehension, and the financial capability to work with a system that is user friendly. But when the deck is stacked against the customer due to low education, poverty, language barrier, or simply the color of one's skin, it often feels like climbing the highest mountain without the necessary tools. According to the International Covenant in Economic, Social, and Cultural Rights, better known as ICESCR, "Access to health care is determined by the availability, accessibility of services to the public; the acceptability to different cultures, sexes, and age groups; and the quality of the services."

So, where do we go from here to equal access and utilization of quality care for not only the forty-seven million uninsured Americans, but also the approximately twenty-five million who are underinsured? The federal government has set a goal of eliminating racial disparities in health care by 2010. But we cannot just sit on the sideline and hope that systemic barriers against minority health care professionals and against minority patients will suddenly disappear. Through blood, sweats, tears, and many lost lives, the Civil Rights era brought about the most profound structural changes in twentieth century American health care system. But there is still enormous unfinished business.

One remark that resonated with me and that I want to share because it rings true today was made in 2003 by Donna Christensen, the U.S delegate from the Virgin Islands: "Before this day is ended, over two hundred African Americans and other people of color will become new casualties in the unacknowledged war against the health of people of color. It appears that this is a war which this country has waged for over forty years—by commission or omission". This was said at a hearing in Chicago, home of our first black president. The numbers might have dwindled slightly to maybe 122 deaths daily, but despite substantial scientific and technological advances in health care over the past decade, a large segment of the American population has not fully benefited from those advances. Disparities apply to a broad array of diseases and an expansive number of life- saving interventions, which many take for granted but are often unavailable to minorities such as angioplasty, advanced treatment for HIV/AIDS, chemotherapy treatments, kidney transplantation, and coronary artery bypass graft surgery. The evidence is clear, consistent, and robust. It is inconceivable that in twenty-first century America, the land of freedom and democracy, so many are aware of the severe and persistent racial inequalities in health care and yet do very little to change these racist practices.

How and why does racism operate so freely? A system of ideologies, policies, and practices is securely in place to perpetuate exclusion and unequal treatment based on race and ethnicity. Fundamental misunderstanding by corporate media underscores this centuries old practice. The impact is also diminished when the word *perceived* is used. It should not be reported as perceived, but instead as what it is: racism. Systemic racism permeates the health care system.

REFERENCES

American Academy of Nursing. (1992). AAN expert panel report: Culturally competent health care. *Nursing Outlook, 4*(6), 277-283.

Anderson, K. L. (2004). Teaching cultural competence using an examplar from literary journalism. *Journal of Nursing Education, 43*, 253-259.

Betancourt, J. R., Green, A. R., & Carrillo, J. E. (2002). *Cultural competence in health care: Emerging frameworks and practical approaches.* New York, NY: The Commonwealth Fund.

Brown, G. (2001). Culture and diversity in the nursing classroom: An impact on communication, *Journal of Cultural Diversity, 8*(1), 16-20.

Bucher, R. D. (2000). *Diversity consciousness: Opening our minds to people, cultures   and opportunity.* Upper Saddle River, NJ: Prentice-Hall.

Bureau of Health Professions. (2002). *Programs to increase diversity.* Washington DC: US Department of Health and Human Services, Health Resources and Services Administration.

Campinha-Bacote, J. (1998). *The process of cultural competence in the delivery of health care services: A culturally competent model of care* (2nd ed.). Cincinnati, OH: Transcultural C.A.R.E Associates.

Campinha-Bacote, J. (2002). The process of cultural competence in the delivery of health care services: A model of care. *Journal of Transcultural Nursing, 13*(3), 181-184.

Campinha-Bacote, J. (2007). *The journey continues* (5th ed.). Cincinnati, OH: Transcultural C.A.R.E associates.

Chan, A. S. (2005). Policy discourses and changing practice: Diversity and the university-college. *Higher Education, 50,* 129-157.

Cowan, D. T., & Norman, I. (2006). Cultural competence in nursing: New meanings. *Journal of Transcultural Nursing, 17,* 102-106.

Institute of Medicine (IOM). (2003). *Unequal Treatment: Confronting racial and ethnic disparities in healthcare.* Washington D.C: National Academy Press.

Office of Minority Health (DHSS, HRSA), (2002). *The National Leadership Summit on Eliminating Racial and Ethnic Disparities in Health.* Washington DC: July 10-12.

Pinar, W. (2001). The gender of racial politics and politics and violence in America: Lynching, prison, rape, and the crisis of masculinity. New York: Peter Long

Porter, C. P., & Barbee, E. (2004). Race and racism in nursing research: Past, present, and future. *Annual Review of Nursing Research, 22,* 9-27.

RAND (2004). Global shift in population: Population matters policy brief. Retrieved August 8, 2008 from www.rand.org/populations/RB/RB5004/

Semmes, C. E. (1996). *Racism, health, and post-industrialism.* Westport, CT: Praeger

U.S Department of Health and Human Services (2000). *Tracking Healthy People 2010.* Washington D.C; US Government Printing Office.

A right delayed is a right denied.

Martin Luther King, Jr.

CHAPTER 4
REFORM TO ELIMINATE RACISM

Health care racism is often unrecognized by the very people who practice it. Although education and health care share the same predicament, they are in many ways so different. Those who avail themselves of these services—parents and students on the one hand, patients and advocates on the other—demand quality and the type of product that a complex systems business model should deliver successfully. Those who provide the services-- teachers, nurses, and doctors-- share these same beliefs and want to provide quality. Unfortunately, the complex systems model is not scalable to the needs of a large society. The only model that scales is the volume operations model which transforms unique relationships into standardized transactions. It is not driven to achieve excellence but rather to meet minimum quality standards as economically as possible.

To succeed at health care reform, one must understand the complexity of the American health care system. The health care system functions much like complex adaptive systems which are distinct from mechanical or electrical complicated systems. A pervasive health policy mistake for many years has been to consider health care systems as complicated when they are, in fact, complex. Many efforts at health care reform consider health care systems and organizations to be built the same way as a computer or a car. If all the pieces can be put together properly, then the system will function well. Complex systems are extremely sensitive to changing conditions. Because health care systems are complex, it is not possible to develop effective formulaic recipes for predictable changes in them. Reform can easily bring about chaos in complex systems like health care. Among the principles of chaos theory is the belief that "a small change in input can quickly translate into overwhelming differences in output." The health care system, due to its magnitude of interconnectedness is extremely sensitive to even the slightest of deviations. This may be the reason why we have this widespread resistance to change. Yet efforts to find set structural answers persist.

Health care is a complex system that has many independent agents who interact with each others. Sometimes they produce change, but for the most part, they create complex adaptive systems containing emergent properties potential. They contain fundamental problems that often lead to famous paradoxes. Very often a distinction is drawn between complex adaptive systems and complex evolving systems. In the former, agents continuously adapt to the changes around them but do not learn from the process. In the latter, agents learn and evolve from each change, thus enabling them to influence their environment, better predict likely changes in the future, and preparing for the challenges. How the various players in a system connect and relate to each another is critical to the survival of the system. The interconnectedness between the players is more important than the players themselves.

Medical care today depends on the interactions between many different individuals participating in all the various parts of the health care system. Knowledge of complexity is central to improving the quality and safety of care. Medical errors arise because of system failure. One example of failure is ineffective collaboration and communication between care providers. This can also be seen in other social systems. The operations of some systems are predictable: repetitive, uniform, and nested. In health care, one needs to reduce unpredictability that leads to failure by implementing simple systems and incorporating their basic qualities. When considering the application of a system to innovative programs, it is important to realize the role of each part and the need to eliminate the parts that are not making positive contributions to the whole.

Systems theory should be implemented with one goal in mind: to increase the effectiveness and efficiency of the total system through the development of manageable subsystems with common focuses or purposes. The subsystem needs to be synchronized, to settle conflicts, and to relate the total organization to its environment. A shared vision among all the major players is required. There has to be a desire for cohesiveness which requires executive leadership to assume new roles and master new skills.

To remain an open and viable system, health care must embrace transparent evaluation and feedback. We need to envision a health care system where every person has similar access regardless of class, income, or status. In the twenty-first century, the health care system faces many challenges, although President George W. Bush saw it as "the best health care system in the world." Furthermore, many Americans are firmly under the illusion that it is the best in the world. Given the amount of money that is swallowed every year by this giant of a system, statements that U.S health care is the best should ring true. But the disturbing truth is that in terms of access to and delivery quality care, the American health care system lags well behind other advanced nations. The World Health Organization was greatly criticized when its report ranked the United States thirty-seventh out of 191 countries, placing it between Costa Rica and Slovenia. A more recent report by the highly regarded Commonwealth Fund ranked the United States last or next-to-last on most measures of performance compared with five other nations: Australia, Canada, Germany, New Zealand and the United Kingdom.

The United States ranks dead last on almost all measures of equity showing the greatest disparity in the quality of care given to richer and poorer citizens. This is surely a measure of incompetence and mismanagement because the world's most powerful economy should be able to provide its citizens with a health care system that not only reflects the best performance the best but should also be a model to others. When its citizens are most vulnerable, they should expect to be treated with the utmost respect and dignity. This is not a question of basic rights, as much as basic human rights.

To explain the dauntingly massive, multi-faceted, all-encompassing reach of the U.S. health care system, Everett Page pointed to the term *reification* which means regarding something abstract as a physical, material thing. "Health care", he said, "is a living, breathing organism, a giant anthropomorphous creature that crawls across the nation, constantly consuming and growing and swelling. Picture an overweight komodo dragon towering over the country, flicking its forked tongue and getting bigger every second. That's health care." The arguments against reform will be the same as always: cost, inefficiency, heavy-handed government control and interference. Race, of course, will never be mentioned as a reason to water down or shelve president Barack Obama's plan. But, as always, it will lurk underneath.

Medicare, a program upon which forty-five million elderly and disabled Americans depend for their health care is fraught with mismanagement and fraud. The U. S government has an annual expenditure of more than $2 trillion on healthcare. On average, at least $70 billion is lost to fraud every year. The anti fraud budget for Medicare is $465 billion a year. According to the U.S Office of Management and Budget's 2008 report, Medicare and Medicaid made improper payments of $23.7 billion in 2007 alone to fraudulent claimants. In South Florida alone, Medicare and Medicaid lost an estimated $ 2.5 billion annually to fraudulent claims. There are statistical disagreements over how big the problem really is. But all will agree that fraud spells bad news for the health care system because it raises healthcare costs for everyone. Higher medical costs, in turn, mean that fewer people can gain access to the healthcare that they need.

Elaborate scams operations bill Medicare for bogus HIV and cancer infusion drugs using dozens of storefronts in Florida, North Carolina, South Carolina, Georgia and Louisiana every year. Early this year, U.S. Attorney General Eric Holder announced the federal government would step up health care antifraud efforts nationally, increasing the budget by 50 percent to $311 million in 2010 and adding manpower to task forces in Miami, Los Angeles, Houston and Detroit. Regarding recent indictments for fraud and the Health Care Fraud Prevention and Enforcement Action Team (HEAT) task force, Department of Health and Human Services Secretary Kathleen Sebelius stated "The Obama administration is committed to turning up the heat on Medicare fraud and employing all the weapons in the federal government's arsenal to target those who are defrauding the American taxpayer. Thanks to cooperation from across the government and some of the best law enforcement professionals in the country, today we were able to save millions of dollars from being lost to criminals and send a powerful message to those who seek to defraud the system that we are coming after them. But our joint efforts on HEAT don't just stop at the jailhouse door. Our Medicare program is working closely in partnership with our own and other law enforcement operations to prevent fraud from happening in the first place. Every dollar we can save by stopping fraud can be used to strengthen the long-term fiscal health of Medicare, bring down costs and deliver better service to Medicare beneficiaries."

Medicare currently pays between 55 and 85 percent more for patented drugs than other government-run health care systems, and pre-tax profit margins on pharmaceuticals in the United States are estimated to be four times larger than those in regulated markets like Canada and the EU (Congressional Budget Office 2004, Vernon 2005). Medicaid fraud diverts valuable health care resources away from those who truly need them. Dishonest providers jeopardize the delivery of quality health care for our elderly, disabled, and poor Americans. Medicare is estimated to remain solvent only until 2018, but experts are optimistic that preventing just 25 percent of the annual combined fraud in Medicare and Medicaid combined fraud can extend the program by at least another ten years. It is therefore obvious that fighting fraud will go a long way toward having the funds needed to reform healthcare. Healthcare is a priority for President Obama and a promise that he must keep to less fortunate Americans. Medicaid and Medicare programs must be reformed to restructure eligibility requirements, especially for the elderly and disabled, so that their benefit allocations are more closely related to their medical needs rather than their socioeconomic status alone. Following are some of the recommendations that have been put forth by health care experts are cited below:

- Reform Medicaid and Medicare programs so that provider compensation is tied to severity of illness and co-morbidity.
- Hold Congressional hearings on racial bias and the impact of racism in health care in America.

- Establish a national presidential and/or congressional advisory committee on racial bias and ethnic health disparities. It should report annually on the status of health care parity to the president and/or Congress through consolidated reports to the Department of Health and Human Services from the Council of Graduate Medical Education, the National Institutes of Health, and the Office of Minority Health.

- Require the American Association of Health Plans, the Joint Commission on Accreditation of Health Care Organizations, the National Committee on Quality Assurance, and other accrediting agencies including those at the state level to adopt uniform standards to collect health care outcome data based on race and ethnicity. These standards should include data on health care participants and providers and should take into account severity of illness, patient confidentiality, methods of collection, and nondiscriminatory use of the data.

According to the National Coalition on Health Care, every thirty seconds an American files for bankruptcy because of a serious health problem. The United States has no comprehensive national health insurance system. Those who have insurance get it through their employers, government programs, or private suppliers. Millions more are underinsured, which has led to the growing epidemic of medical debt and bankruptcy in the United States

There are some common sense recommendations for reform that have been discussed by everyone in the know. I hope that the president's advisors have been listening.

- Increase the availability of generic drugs. Low-cost generic drugs could save Medicare, Medicaid and consumers billions of dollars.
- Close the loopholes that allow drug makers to hold on to their patents and slow the introduction of generic drugs to the market. Businesses and the government should use their combined buying power to negotiate lower drug prices. The pharmaceutical companies will, of course resist this, but it will be of immense benefits to the public and will save hundred of millions of dollars for the government.
- Increase transparency and accountability for Pharmacy Benefit Managers (PBMs), third party administrators, who negotiate deals with drug makers on behalf of insurers, state health programs, and large businesses. These deals are shrouded in secrecy. Many plaintiffs who have brought lawsuits against the PBMs have alleged that they fail to act in their clients' best fiduciary interest.

The Food and Drug Administration (FDA) has sent many notices to drug companies warning that the marketing for over one hundred different drugs was false and/or misleading; nonetheless such practices persist. More than once the FDA has reprimanded many of the leading pharmaceutical companies for misrepresented risks and misleading claims. Drug marketing is pervasive, dangerous, and aimed primarily at doctors, a benign relationship that starts as early as medical school. Everyday the media bombards the general public with drug advertisement. This practice should be banned because it has been proven to have great influence on decisions related to prescribing medication.

The government should set up an action committee to investigate deceptive marketing and create federal and state guidelines for doctors to have access to independent and accurate information about drugs. The information produced by the clinical trial registry should be packaged by an independent group or agency into a form easily usable by prescribers who want information about treatment options. This is currently available but it is aimed more at policymakers than prescribers.

Bureaucrats and lobbyists of the pharmaceutical companies will argue that although the use of prescription drugs is on the increase in the United States, the cost of prescription medications represents just over ten cents of every dollar spent. Americans spend over $285 billion annually on prescription drugs; reducing the cost to five cents on every dollar will yield savings in the millions. The rank and file in the pharmaceutical industry might consider millions of dollars to be might insignificant, but a few million here and there are worth plenty and will count toward the new health care reform. The U.S. pharmaceutical industry has agreed to spend $80 billion over the next ten years to reduce drug costs for seniors and help pay for President Obama's proposed health care reform plan. They should be asked to double the amount to at least $160 billion. That would be a fair price for a place at the table.

A similar approach should be applied to the insurance companies. To date, they have not offered to pay for anything from their king- size profits. Just applying a simple levy on the pharmaceutical and insurance companies will put $32 billions a year in the coffers. This can be directed toward the $63.5 billion a year that the president has earmarked to help finance reform of our health care system to bring down costs, expand coverage, and improve quality.

This is an honest discussion that we need to have in America today. Pumping more money into the health care system does not necessarily change attitudes. In view of the hundreds of already published studies showing health care disparities there should be meetings and debates in town halls and universities with our president, a man of color and our chief health care reformer. Reform should start at the base instead of at the top of the iceberg. This book is not revealing alarming new discoveries. It is trying to consolidate in very plain and simple language information that already exists in lengthy documents, books, dissertations, and researches. But because they are lengthy and often geared towards academia, findings are not read by the vast majority of concerned Americans.

Simply put, there are more than 255 million Americans who currently are very fortunate to have insurance. We therefore have this pervasive feeling that most are covered and too bad for the rest! Many people who are insured are not willing to enter into a health reform program that could potentially affect their access to a doctor. Why should they be worried or concerned about the 47 million who are uninsured? They should each take a deep breath and realize that they are but a paycheck away from loosing a job, and with it their health coverage.

The uninsured are not necessarily unemployed or unwilling to work. Eighty percent of the uninsured are small business owners or those who have been obliged to take early retirement without insurance benefits. Findings from the 2004 census reveal that recent increases in the number of uninsured or underinsured include working Americans who were declined employee-sponsored health insurance. These are hard- working individuals making an annual salary of $30,000 to $50,000 who just cannot afford to buy insurance coverage for themselves and their families.

Many of the low income minority employees are eligible for Medicaid or the CHIP program, but they are unaware that they can qualify or are eligible. They often find the enrollment process daunting. These are full- time or part- time workers in low paying jobs or workers in transition between jobs. This category alone accounts for approximately ten million Americans. When this problem is raised for discussion, it always brings out the worse in many of the "haves." They are ready to introduce the scare tactics of rationing, affordability, and government take-over.

Most of the large corporations use your health care coverage as the carrot to keep employees on board until the time they are no longer needed or can be replaced by cheaper labor. In order for most Americans to support major changes, more Americans will have to lose their employer-based insurance coverage and be forced to search for individual coverage. That might come soon enough. The Bureau of the Census reported that more than one million fewer Americans were covered by employer-based insurance in 2007 compared to 2006. If that number continues to grow over the next five years, the United States may reach the tipping point when enough people will push for major changes. And be aware that over the past three years more than six hundred thousand Americans have found themselves unemployed and uninsured. Have we become so self- absorbed and consumed by our own priorities that we have lost sight of those less fortunate?

Another extremely weak argument against reform is that if a public option plan is approved there will not be enough doctors to care for the forty-seven million uninsured who will gain access and utilization to the system. The truth is that a public option will force the health industry to redesign care placing the patient at the center with a doctor (such as a primary care physician) to coordinate relevant care with the help of nurse- practitioners, preferably minority nurse practitioners. This will boost the number of racially diverse doctors and nurses and firmly set up health care providers on the road to cultural competence. What a win-win situation for patients and care givers in the twenty-first century!

The biggest advantage of a public health insurance option serves two essential goals of health care reform. First, it will provide needed competition in places where a single private insurer currently dominate the market and hold the consumer hostage. Second, if the private insurers' size and profit are reduced, its clout will be diminished allowing others to compete, creating a fairer market, and the market and leveling the playing field. After all, that, fairness and competition are the basic tenets of the American market, not monopoly.

These very attributes have earned the public option the wrath of the insurance, pharmaceutical, and hospital industries, even as it remains the most promising vehicle for driving down health care costs. President Obama and his team, eager for a compromise, have begun downplaying the necessity of a public plan as the pillar of a reformed health system. Of the many goals of health care reform, bringing down costs is the most obvious benefit for all Americans. A public plan would achieve savings from not only its bargaining power but also its lack of dividends and exorbitant private-sector executive salaries. Competition with a public plan would force private insurers to reduce costs and adhere strictly to regulations forbidding insurers from excluding customers with preexisting conditions or charging them higher rates. Those were the promises that Barack Obama made on the campaign trail and those are the very concepts that are worth fighting for. After nearly fifty years in the making, they will be considered real reform.

At a speech made on October 23, 2009, to colleagues at the University of California, San Francisco, Dr. Rodgers, an expert on health care disparities, delivered a heartfelt message: "It goes without saying that the disproportionate number of blacks and Hispanics who lack adequate health insurance contributes to health care disparities," she said. "Universal coverage is critically important but not adequate to solving the problem of health disparities. During this critical time in our nation's history it is critically important that we all do our part in helping our elected leaders understand the importance of universal coverage with a public option until we can get to single payer. All of us interested in eliminating health disparities must be willing to move away from the comfortable walls of academia and speak our truths about the adverse health consequences of racism, sexism, homophobia, and poverty."

In a fact sheet released in March 2009, the Families USA's Minority Health Initiative made available some startling figures: "Almost half (45.8 percent) of people of color under the age of sixty-five went without health coverage for some or all of the two-year period 2007-2008. The numbers were even more alarming when broken down by race and ethnicity: more than half of Hispanics/Latinos (55.1 percent), two out of five African Americans (40.3 percent), and one-third of other racial and ethnic minorities2 (34 percent) were uninsured, compared to one-quarter of whites (25.8 percent)."

It is very fitting to conclude this chapter by two quotes. Dr Tommy Thompson, former secretary of Health and Human Services stated "Communities of color suffer disproportionately from diabetes, heart disease, HIV/AIDS, cancer, stroke, and infant mortality. Eliminating these and other health disparities is a priority of HHS". The second quote is from former Senator Bill Frist (R- TN) when he was majority leader. Regarding his priorities for the 108th Congress, he stated "We need to focus on the uninsured and those who suffer from health care disparities".

REFERENCES

Arrow, K. et al (209). Towards a 21ˢᵗ Century Health Care System: Recommendations for Health Care Reform. *Annals of Internal Medicine, 150(7)*: 493—495.

Byrd W. M., & Clayton, L. (2000). *An American Health Dilemma.* Volume I. New York: Routledge.

Coffman, J. M. et al. Racial /Ethnic Disparities in Nursing. *Health Affairs*, May 2001.

CBS News—60 minutes (209). Medicare Fraud: A $60 Billion Crime.

James, S. A. (2003). Confronting the Moral Econoy of US Racial/Ethnic Health Disparities. *American Journal of Public Health, 93(2):* 189.

Mangano, M. F. Principal Deputy Inspector General, U.S. Department of Health and Human Services. *Testimony on Fraud in Medicare Programs. (*Before the Senate Committee on Governmental Affairs).

McKethan, A. et al (2009*). Improving Quality and Value in the U.S Health Care System.* Brookings Institute.

For the great enemy of the truth is very often not the lie—deliberate, contrived and dishonest—but the myth, persistent, persuasive, and unrealistic. Too often we hold fast to the clichés of our forebears. We subject all facts to a prefabricated set of interpretations. We enjoy the comfort of opinion without the discomfort of thought.

John F. Kennedy.

CHAPTER 5
RECOMMENDATIONS

For over forty years in America, a successful government run plan called Medicare has offered universal coverage to millions of disabled Americans and those over age sixty-five. While it has its flaws because of the billions of dollars in mismanaged funds and the huge bureaucracy needed to oversee it, Medicare can provide a valuable lesson if we can all take the time to analyze its many advantages and recognize its failures. The downfalls are mainly due to a health care system that has expanded unchecked, similar to many infrastructures built in a different era and unable to cope with demands and technologies of the twenty-first centuries. We cannot expect a nineteenth century system to still be relevant today. Medicare should be reorganized from a fee- for- service reimbursement to a quality and results reimbursement model.

A huge part of Medicare is a gift to the insurance industry to the tune of $175 billions a year. The insurance companies never intended to be good faith partners. The insurance companies have long been major stakeholders in the health care industry. They have always been completely self- serving. Their efforts to eliminate high risk consumers, especially those with pre- existing conditions, from the insurance pools and their total disregard for the health care of the underprivileged should be a focus of lawmakers on Capitol Hill. They have put up smoke screens to pretend that they will be willing to restructure. But all along the Health Insurance Association of America, founded in 1956, has spent millions to create fearmongering advertisements to scare the public.

Many in the insurance industry like angels of doom waiting to prey on the feeble and the sick. They are against competing in a fair marketplace. Integrity and transparency are not part of the strategies to bring equality and equity. From price gouging to collusion, the insurance industry has been allowed to operate in a manner that no other financial service sector can because they are exempt by the anti trust laws. They need to be forced by the government to get on board for true reform: to renegotiate drug prices, to remove pre existing conditions and lifetime caps, and to increase portability.

Americans do not need misaligned incentives. Politics always seem to triumph over relevant policies in Congress. Americans today do not need a diluted form of health care reform. Since 17 percent of the U.S economy already goes to keep health care afloat, cost containment, affordability, and equality of care should be part of the health care package. Entrenched bureaucracy that favors the status of employer-based insurance and the monopoly of the insurance companies must be overturned. The American people must be made aware, in simple language minus the rhetoric, that 94 to 98 percent of the insurance market is not competitive due to the stranglehold by one or two powerful insurance companies. That is communism at its best...and the fear mongers are so apt to use the "socialist" bogeyman!

I recently read an article about integrated systems in health care that contain costs while maintaining quality. That sounds to me like a winner. Gundersen Lutheran, a health care system in western Wisconsin has the fourth-lowest health care costs in the country based on Medicare spending. It employs over 6000 workers of which over 450 are physicians. What they are doing, and have been doing so successfully I might add is proof that the United States can slow the rise in health care spending without hurting quality.

Many challenge the contention that slowing the rise in health care spending will mean denying patients needed care. They refute the widely held belief that more care is better care, and that expensive care is even better. This is the old way of thinking and it is not based on evidence but on fear of change and commitment to retaining the status quo. Better results can be obtained by eliminating duplicative and unnecessary care, preventing illness or detecting it earlier, avoiding unneeded or preventable hospitalizations, increasing productivity and reducing administrative costs. These are things that have been tried and proven extremely successful.

Unfortunately, only a few health systems have tried them. No simple explanation exists why Gundersen Lutheran or the Mayo Health System can provide quality care at a fraction of the cost of their counterparts in California, Miami or Texas. Lutheran and Mayo are integrated health care systems that employ doctors, and research suggests that integrated systems and large physician practices closely aligned with a hospital often produce better care at a lower cost. One of the points discussed was that doctors run the health system. The doctors are expected to become involved in its operations and to work to control costs. They are well paid and make an excellent living. They just aren't the highest paid. The doctors at Gundersen Lutheran repeatedly refer to the value placed on cooperation and on a focus on the patient. Integrated health system work to recruit doctors who understand those values.

Integration gives Gundersen Lutheran a huge advantage in coordinating care, getting information on best practices to physicians and creating a culture of shared values, said Thompson, its chief executive. The health system's orthopedic surgeons, for example, reduced costs by $900,000 a year just by getting together and agreeing to use medical devices from one supplier. Standardizing care also is easier in an integrated system. The doctors at Gundersen Lutheran have developed specific guidelines and order sets for specific diseases and procedures. The challenge is how to make the U.S. health care system look more like Gundersen Lutheran and other integrated systems. The challenge is how to make the U.S. health care system look more like Gundersen Lutheran and other integrated systems. Integration is not the norm in the U.S. health care system.

As recently as 2005, roughly half of all office visits were made to practices with one or two physicians, according to the National Ambulatory Medical Care Survey. There is a higher percentage of physicians in one or two-person practices. That kind of fragmentation is characteristic of the U.S. health care system, and it is one of the challenges in slowing the growth in health care spending. Even a slight reduction of 1.5 percent in the projected rise in health care spending could save trillions of dollars over ten years. These savings translate into millions more disenfranchised Americans receiving quality health care.

The high cost of technological innovation in the health care industry is one of the primary reasons for driving prices up. First, health care is one of our most basic needs and, as such, the idea of a market segmented by willingness to pay, in which some patients receive a lower standard of care, violates social norms as well as individuals' preferences for their own care. Second, as previously mentioned the 225 millions Americans with insurance bear such a small fraction of their costs out of pocket that they are largely insensitive to price. They unfortunately do not realize how fragile that security net of employer based health insurance is. Thirdly, health care consumers typically often blindly follow the advice of their physicians rather than make their own value-based trade-offs about their treatment. This usually amount to billions of dollars in unnecessary tests and medications. Finally, there is a scarcity of quality comparisons among treatments that would allow patients or physicians to make value-based comparisons of the treatment options.

Adding to the problem is fee-for-service reimbursement, the predominant payment method for outpatient care which requires care providers to bear little of the risk of patient treatment. In fact, fee-for-service creates strong financial incentives for care givers to offer more, and more costly care to patients. More visits, more tests, more procedures all add up to more cost. A simple in-office visit and an X-ray usually cost about $125. If the doctor adds an MRI performed in-office or within the same physician practice, the cost goes up to $500 in professional fees and a $350 facility fee.

Because doctors largely determine most courses of treatment, the combination of fee-for-service reimbursement and the practice of defensive medicine to avoid any malpractice suits reinforce comprehensive approaches to care. It is at the physician's discretion whether a simple in-office examination is sufficient or whether more diagnostic tests such as X-rays, CT scans, or MRIs should be conducted to confirm the findings of a physical examination. While research suggests that the direct costs of malpractice lawsuits are limited, an average of $60 billion a year, the risk of litigation creates an incentive for doctors to err on the side of caution. Precautionary tests limit a doctor's personal risks while at the same time generate higher reimbursements when treating any individual patient. In the end, all contribute to the cost of health care spiraling out of control.

The simplest recommendation is that general access to quality care can increase utilization and prevent delay in seeking care.

According to many researchers, access to health care decreases chronic illnesses and increase life expectancy. Unfortunately, due to subpar coverage or lack of insurance, minorities have greater difficulty accessing health care services. Therefore cooler heads and a more careful assessments of the present system must prevail to convince opponents to health care reform that, if done right, there will be great benefits to minorities who earn lower wages and to the unemployed who are unable to obtain health insurance.

By health care reform, I do not mean mandating that everyone buy insurance or be penalized. Some people, with or without health care reform will still not be able to afford the cost. Large numbers of middle- class working Americans cannot afford it now. Real health care reform is asking two basic questions: (1) Why do we keeping a system that allows twenty thousand people to die each year from limited access to the system? (2) Why do we allow the top ten insurance company executives to receive $690 million in bonuses in an industry that provides no value to health?

Cost containment should start with the implementation of a voucher system for those between twenty-one and thirty-one years of age, and for those still in college. The fact that many minority patients obtain non-urgent care in emergency department has been well documented. According to the National Ambulatory Medical Care Survey, more than sixty million emergency department visits yearly are for non-urgent care by those who are uninsured. In general, an emergency room visit is more expensive than comparable care received in a physician's office. And if the uninsured patient has to receive any laboratory tests, ultrasound,

X-ray, mammogram, MRI, CT scan, EKG, vaccination, anesthesia, or other miscellaneous diagnostic procedures, the final bill, ultimately paid by those with insurance, is astronomical. "Emergency departments are a "safety net" and often the place of first resort for health care for America's poor and uninsured," according to Linda McCaig of the CDC's National Center for Health Statistics said in a statement. A very expensive safety net, I might add: $120 million a year to be exact!!

The real safety nets are the Community Health Centers. For more than forty years, these Health Centers have provided comprehensive, culturally competent, and quality care to the uninsured and the underserved. The centers have been the backbone of the primary care safety net in the United States since the 1960s. They are a product of the Civil Rights movement to provide accessible health care to low income or unemployed Americans. The Community Health Centers are mandated by Congress to provide care to minorities, the homeless, those not able to speak English, and the migrant workers who would otherwise be without health care.

In 2009, approximately forty percent of patients care for at the Community Health Centers were 19 years of age and younger. The number of patients across America who received care at the Centers are estimated at eight millions. Because they care for such a vulnerable group of patients, these Health Centers should be earmarked for more funds from the government as they are providing a substantial amount of care. In reality, these safety nets face a complex set of challenges. It is doubtful that health care reform done half heartedly will increase support for these safety nets. However, if policymakers are truly interested in equal treatment for all Americans, they should examine in details how these Community Health Centers are able to provide high quality, "disparity-free" services to persons of color and other racial and ethnic patients. Reform, depending on its final structure, may hopefully strengthen the safety nets' ability to continue their valuable work.

It is clear that to be effective any action implemented in the future must address each of the drivers of cost, quality, and access. To realize such a tall order, it will be necessary to manage demand while ensuring that supply keeps pace with demand. The United States also needs to address the financing of health care and ensure that any reform take place within an effective organizationl. To manage demand for health care products and services, the health care system needs to work hard on the two levers of preventing illness and ensuring that consumers or purchasers of health care become valueconscious. The role of payers, employers, and the government must be to promote innovation that will decrease costs and improve quality.

The three basic problems of our current system are like the three legs of a stool. Cost, quality, and access must be tackled as a package. Tinkering with one while ignoring the others will never bring about positive outcomes. Improving access for low income Americans and those on Medicare and Medicaid while ignoring cost containment will be disastrous to the survival of the system. On the other hand cost containment without a logical long- term plan will be totally detrimental to quality and access, especially to minorities who are already being short-changed on both access and quality of care. Policymakers and Congress agree that cost must be contained, but they disagree on how to really tame this beast. Some think that there need to be a strict price and budget control on health care spending. Others believe that free market competition is the solution.

The optimal approach to stop or slow cost inflation across the health care supply chain is to prevent overconsumption of services by an ever increasing exigent consumer who are not fully cognizant of the damaging effect of their gluttony on the system. Many of the demands on the system are really due to chronic conditions. It all starts from unhealthy lifestyles, unavailability of healthy food, and no access to early care. Such tragic combinations are costly in the long run. Such chronic conditions as hypertension, diabetes, kidney failure, and heart disease are high cost tickets for the health care system.

Prevention, restraint from instant gratification, and a radical change in lifestyle are needed now. But most Americans are addicted to high processed food that is readily available and cheap. It also tastes good and keeps addicted people happy. With instant happiness comes a lifetime of consequences. Heavy taxes must be placed on such items alcohol, tobacco, sodas, sugary and salty snacks, and all the extra costs associated with obesity. This epidemic of unhealthy Americans is not being seriously evaluated. This is accumulated credit that will need to be paid at a hefty price compounded by years of interest by a health care system already overburdened.

In addition to issues of supply and demand, health care intermediaries need to promote sustainable financing mechanisms to collect and distribute funds. Within the context of the principal issues we have discussed, policy makers must determine the most effective financing and payment approach to align provider incentives with giving an appropriate amount and type of care. More is not always better. As the stakeholders in the US health system attempt to answer these critical questions, we see four broad approaches to implementation of reform, which appear along a spectrum from indirect to direct interventions. Public awareness must be raised to the benefits of prevention and healthy lifestyles. Appropriate incentives must be created, desired behavior must be mandated, and direct action must be taken to achieve the desired results.

REFERENCE

Coddington, D. C. (1990). The Crisis in Health Care: Costs, choices, and strategies. Jossey—Bass, San Francisco.

Committee on the Consequences of Uninsurance, Board on Health Care Services, IOM (2001).

Coverage matters: Insurance and Health care. National Academy Press, Washington DC.

Eisenberg, J.M., & Power, E. J. (2000). Transforming insurance coverage into quality health care:

Voltage drops from potential to delivered quality. *JAMA 284:* 2100—2107.

Feagin, J. R., & McKinney, K.D. (2003). The Many Costs of Racism. Oxfors, MA: Rowman & Littlefield Publishers.

Jones, C. p. (2004). Confronting Institutional Racism. *Phylon*, 7-22.

Marquis, M.S., & Long, S.H. Effects of "second generation" small group health insurance market reforms. *Inquiry, 2001,38*: 365—380.

Nazroo, J. Y. (2003). The Structuring of Ethnic Inequalities in Health: Economic Position, Racial Discrimination, and Racism. *American Journal of Public Health, 93(2):* 277-284.

We must be the change we want to see in the world.

Mahatma Gandhi.

EPILOGUE

I believe that the health care system must provide an adequate organizational framework that ensures the effective implementation of raising public awareness toward the real cost of health care, educating the American public on how unhealthy habits are breeding a future nation of young Americans plagued by diabetes, high blood pressure, and obesity.

Talks of health care reform by president Obama have brought out the worst in those who want him to fail. The rhetoric from both the left and the right, from politicians and activists, has been heated and very misleading. They are jealously guarding a system that is truly substandard and not benefiting the American people. In light of what is being revealed every-day, how can we hope to make the insurance industry honest and transparent? Congressmen on both the right and the left have received millions of dollars in campaign contributions from the insurance industry, an industry that is recession- proof and thriving while 122 Americans die each day from lack of adequate health care. So the insurance companies already have created their own "Death Panels" system!

The current system, insurance based and employment centered are not favored by 70 percent of Americans. Yet some Republicans are inciting hatred and violence and saying that they are not in favor of a public option plan because they do not want a government bureaucrat between the patient and his or her doctor. We all know that most Americans already has an insurance company bureaucrat between them and their doctor-an insurance company bureaucrat whose sole purpose is to deny that person appropriate care if deemed too costly. The American public deserves better than lame and ridiculous excuses.

Why don't we hear the true reason for not passing health care reform? Could it be that about 25 percent of population will do anything in their power to humiliate, obstruct, and defeat the first black president of the United States? As they have proclaimed for centuries, black is inferior and incapable; therefore a black president must be shown to be a failure and incapable of leading this country. Despite helping to bail out the world banking system, saving the world's largest insurer, rescuing the American auto industry and an American sea captain held captive by pirates, passing a stimulus package and a budget in only the first three months of his presidency, he is vilified and blamed day after day unlike his predecessor who received carte blanche to bring this proud country of ours to its knees. George W. Bush was hailed as a patriot and a good Christian. Barack Obama is labeled Un-American, a Nazi, and compared to Hitler. The Obama presidency has been a whirlwind of policymaking and legislation, crisis management and confidence-building, international diplomacy, and cautious management of two existing wars. Such work should be applauded, not denigrated.

Or it is simply that the privileged do not really care about equal access to quality health care for all Americans regardless of race, color, creed, gender or economic status? For true reform to happen we must all embrace key values that will foster a justice-based health care system, thus minimizing inequities in access to quality of care. Every other country in the industrialized world has opted for a not-for-profit health care system. They have long understood that for-profit systems are too costly, complex, unfair, bureaucratic, and inefficient. The model has also proven to be bad for those less fortunate and also extremely detrimental to the economy.

Yes, the president has a full plate, but his priority for this year must be health care reform. Given the growing knowledge of the subtle and complex nature of institutional racism within the health care system, he must bring about reform by neutralizing and eliminating it. He must call for a thorough review of the recruitment and retention of health care professionals, the inadequate number of minority professionals in positions of institutional leadership, andthe harsh, unsupportive, and unwelcoming climate that minority nursing, dental, and medical students must endure in silence.

Today, while African Americans, Hispanics, and Native Americans represent over 32 percent of the population, they constitute less than 11 percent of nurses, 7 percent of physicians, and 6 percent of dentists. Only Asian Americans seem to be well represented in the medical field. This represent a sliver of the actual problem, but a thorough examination must start at the level of the foundation, the very people that will eventually change the face of this system.

The president must be steadfast in his resolve. A victorious person is one who can persevere no matter what. Let us reflect on this quote from Thurgood Marshall and ask ourselves what we want from the health care system of the future: "A child born to a black mother in a state like Mississippi… has exactly the same rights as a white baby born to the wealthiest person in the United States. It's not true, but I challenge anyone to say it is not a goal worth working for."

www.ingramcontent.com/pod-product-compliance
Lightning Source LLC
Chambersburg PA
CBHW072207280526
45788CB00002B/910